Atkins Diet Cookbook For Beginners

Simple, Delicious, and Easy-to-Follow Low-Carb Recipes for Weight Loss And Healthy Living

Emily M. Wilson

Copyright © 2023 Emily M. Wilson

All rights reserved.

No part of this publication may be reproduced, distributed, or transmitted in any form or by any means, including photocopying, recording, or other electronic or mechanical methods, without the prior written permission of the publisher, except in the case of brief quotations embodied in critical reviews and certain other noncommercial uses permitted by copyright law.

Contents

INTRODUCTION 7

    UNDERSTANDING THE ATKINS DIET 7

    HOW THE DIET WORKS 7

    BENEFITS AND CONSIDERATIONS 7

    SHOPPING LIST: STOCKING UP FOR YOUR ATKINS DIET JOURNEY 8

CHAPTER ONE: RECIPES 11

    DELICIOUS BREAKFAST 11

        Avocado and Bacon Breakfast Bowl 11

        Spinach and Mushroom Mini Quiches 12

        Coconut Chia Pudding 13

        Almond Flour Pancakes 14

        Greek Yogurt and Berry Parfait 15

        Smoked Salmon and Cream Cheese Wrap 16

        Green Eggs and Ham Scramble 17

        Keto Breakfast Burrito Bowl 18

        Low-Carb Breakfast Burrito 19

        Cinnamon Walnut Cottage Cheese Bowl 20

    SATISFYING LUNCH 21

        Grilled Chicken Caesar Salad 21

        Turkey Avocado Lettuce Wraps 22

        Zucchini Noodles with Pesto and Cherry Tomatoes 23

        Tuna Salad Lettuce Wraps 24

        Broccoli and Cheddar Stuffed Chicken 25

        Cauliflower Fried Rice 26

        Egg Salad Lettuce Wraps 27

        Beef and Broccoli Stir-Fry 28

        Creamy Avocado Tuna Salad 29

        Mediterranean Chicken Salad 30

NUTRIENT-PACKED DINNER 31

Baked Salmon with Asparagus and Lemon 31

Grilled Steak with Roasted Brussels Sprouts 32

Stuffed Bell Peppers with Ground Turkey 33

Garlic Butter Shrimp and Zoodles 34

Baked Stuffed Portobello Mushrooms 35

Cauliflower Crust Pizza 36

Lemon Herb Grilled Chicken with Steamed Broccoli 37

Spinach and Feta Stuffed Chicken Breast 38

Eggplant Parmesan 39

Beef Stir-Fry with Broccoli and Peppers 40

WHOLESOME SNACK AND APPETIZER 41

Guacamole and Veggie Sticks 41

Deviled Eggs 42

Cucumber and Cream Cheese Bites 43

Almond-Stuffed Dates Wrapped in Bacon 44

Smoked Salmon Cucumber Bites 45

Spicy Buffalo Cauliflower Bites 46

Zucchini Parmesan Crisps 47

Caprese Skewers 48

Mixed Nuts and Cheese Platter 49

SOUPS AND SALADS 51

Mexican Cauliflower Rice Salad 51

Zucchini and Tomato Salad 52

Tomato Basil Soup with Parmesan Crisps 53

Asian Cabbage Salad with Grilled Steak 54

Spicy Chicken and Kale Soup 55

Grilled Shrimp Salad with Lemon Herb Dressing 56

Cauliflower and Leek Soup 58

Greek Salad with Grilled Chicken 59

Creamy Mushroom Soup 60

Cobb Salad with Ranch Dressing ... 61
Roasted Red Pepper and Tomato Soup ... 62
Avocado Cucumber Salad ... 63
Spinach and Strawberry Salad ... 64
Lemon Chicken Orzo Soup ... 65
Zucchini Noodle Salad with Pesto Dressing ... 66

POULTRY AND SEAFOOD RECIPES ... 67

Pesto Grilled Salmon ... 67
Creamy Garlic Parmesan Chicken ... 68
Coconut Lime Grilled Chicken ... 69
Herb-Crusted Baked Cod ... 70
Cajun Grilled Turkey Breast ... 71
Creamy Tuscan Shrimp ... 72
Rosemary Roasted Chicken Thighs ... 73
Seared Tuna Steak with Avocado Salsa ... 74

SIDE DISHES ... 75

Spiced Cabbage and Carrot Slaw ... 75
Broccoli and Almond Stir-Fry ... 76
Garlic Roasted Asparagus ... 77
Cauliflower Mash with Garlic and Chives ... 78
Cabbage and Radish Slaw ... 79
Mushroom and Spinach Sauté ... 80
Roasted Eggplant with Tahini Drizzle ... 81
Green Bean and Cherry Tomato Salad ... 82

VEGETARIAN ENTREES ... 83

Cauliflower and Broccoli Rice Stir-Fry ... 83
Eggplant and Mushroom Ratatouille ... 85
Portobello Mushroom and Goat Cheese Stuffed Squash ... 86
Chickpea and Spinach Coconut Curry ... 87
Spaghetti Squash with Pesto and Roasted Tomatoes ... 88
Brussels Sprouts and Pecan Salad ... 90

Cauliflower and Spinach Curry 91
DESSERT 93
Strawberry Chia Seed Pudding 93
Coconut Lime Panna Cotta 94
Vanilla Ricotta Parfait with Berries 95
Coconut Flour Lemon Bars 96
Almond Butter Chocolate Fudge 97
Pumpkin Spice Cheesecake Bites 98
Mixed Berry Crumble 99
Chocolate Avocado Mousse 100
Coconut Chia Seed Popsicles 101
Raspberry Almond Thumbprint Cookies 102
Cinnamon Almond Baked Apples 103

CHAPTER TWO: 28-DAY MEAL PLAN 105

7-DAY WEIGHT LOSS EXERCISE PLAN 107

CONCLUSION 109

BONUS: WEIGHT LOSS JOURNAL 111

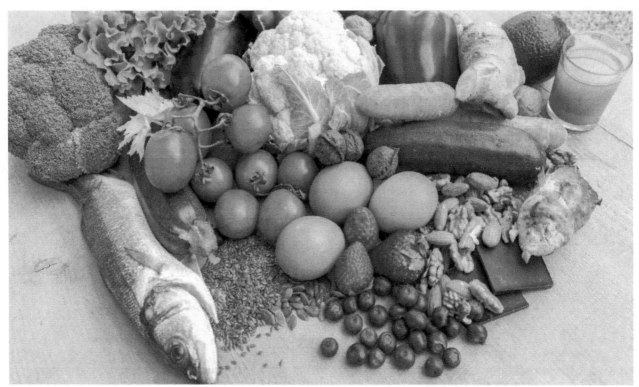

INTRODUCTION

The Atkins Diet, a groundbreaking approach to weight loss and improved health, has captured the attention of individuals seeking a balanced way to shed unwanted pounds and maintain a sustainable lifestyle. Rooted in the vision of Dr. Robert Atkins, a cardiologist who challenged conventional dietary norms, the Atkins Diet reimagines the role of carbohydrates in our daily meals.

UNDERSTANDING THE ATKINS DIET

At its core, the Atkins Diet revolves around the concept that the body's metabolism reacts differently to varying levels of carbohydrate intake. This philosophy challenges the traditional notion that fat is the primary culprit behind weight gain. Instead, the diet places a significant focus on controlling carbohydrate consumption while embracing moderate protein and healthy fat intake. This distinctive approach aims to transition the body into a state of ketosis, where it primarily burns fat for fuel.

HOW THE DIET WORKS

The Atkins Diet is divided into several phases, each designed to ease individuals into a healthier eating pattern and aid in achieving specific weight loss and health goals. The initial phase, Induction, limits carbohydrate intake to a minimum, kickstarting the body's transition into ketosis. As the diet progresses, the Balancing phase introduces a slightly higher carbohydrate intake while maintaining steady weight loss. The Pre-Maintenance and Maintenance phases gradually reintroduce more carbohydrates, promoting weight stability and individualized carbohydrate tolerance.

BENEFITS AND CONSIDERATIONS

Numerous benefits are associated with the Atkins Diet, extending beyond weight loss. Research suggests that reduced carbohydrate intake may lead to improved blood sugar control, reduced triglyceride levels, and increased levels of high-density lipoprotein (HDL) cholesterol.

Additionally, some individuals report enhanced energy levels and reduced cravings for refined sugars and processed foods.

However, like any dietary approach, the Atkins Diet has considerations. Adapting to a lower carbohydrate intake might cause initial discomfort, commonly referred to as the "keto flu," as the body adjusts to burning fat for energy. It's essential to stay hydrated and ensure sufficient intake of fiber-rich vegetables. Individuals with certain medical conditions, such as kidney issues, should consult healthcare professionals before embarking on this diet.

SHOPPING LIST: STOCKING UP FOR YOUR ATKINS DIET JOURNEY

1. **Plan Ahead:** Before heading to the store, take a moment to plan your meals for the upcoming week. This will help you create a focused shopping list and prevent impulse purchases.
2. **Prioritize Protein:** Protein is a cornerstone of the Atkins Diet. Load up on lean meats like chicken, turkey, beef, and fish. Consider adding tofu, eggs, and Greek yogurt for variety.
3. **Embrace Healthy Fats:** Opt for sources of healthy fats like avocados, nuts, seeds, and olive oil. These fats are essential for keeping you satisfied and supporting your body's needs.
4. **Green and Colorful Veggies:** Fill your cart with an assortment of low-carb vegetables such as spinach, kale, broccoli, cauliflower, bell peppers, and zucchini. These veggies are versatile and nutrient-packed.
5. **Low-Carb Fruits:** Choose berries like strawberries, blueberries, and raspberries for a touch of sweetness without the excess sugar. Limit higher-carb fruits like bananas and grapes.
6. **Dairy Choices:** Look for full-fat dairy products like cheese, cream, and unsweetened Greek yogurt. These options fit well within the Atkins Diet's parameters.
7. **Low-Carb Pantry Staples:** Stock up on essentials like almond flour, coconut flour, psyllium husk, and sugar substitutes for baking and cooking.

8. **Read Labels:** When purchasing packaged foods, read the nutrition labels carefully to ensure they fit your low-carb requirements. Pay attention to serving sizes and hidden sugars.
9. **Stay Hydrated:** Don't forget to include beverages like herbal tea, sparkling water, and water enhancers on your list to stay hydrated without added sugars.
10. **Snack Wisely:** Include snacks that align with your Atkins Diet goals, such as nuts, seeds, jerky, and low-carb protein bars. Having these on hand can help you avoid temptations.
11. **Spices and Herbs:** Enhance the flavor of your meals with a variety of herbs and spices. They can make low-carb dishes exciting and satisfying.
12. **Frozen and Canned Options:** Consider frozen vegetables, seafood, and lean meats for longer shelf life. Canned options like tuna, salmon, and vegetables can also be handy.
13. **Batch Cooking Ingredients:** If you plan to meal prep, buy ingredients in bulk to save money and time. Cook and freeze large portions for convenience.
14. **Stick to the List:** While at the store, focus on purchasing items from your prepared shopping list. This helps prevent impulse purchases that might not align with your diet goals.
15. **Stay Open to New Foods:** The Atkins Diet encourages exploration. Be open to trying new low-carb foods and recipes to keep your meals exciting and diverse.

Remember, successful shopping is a vital step toward your Atkins Diet journey. By being mindful of your choices and prioritizing nutrient-rich foods, you're setting yourself up for a satisfying and sustainable way of eating.

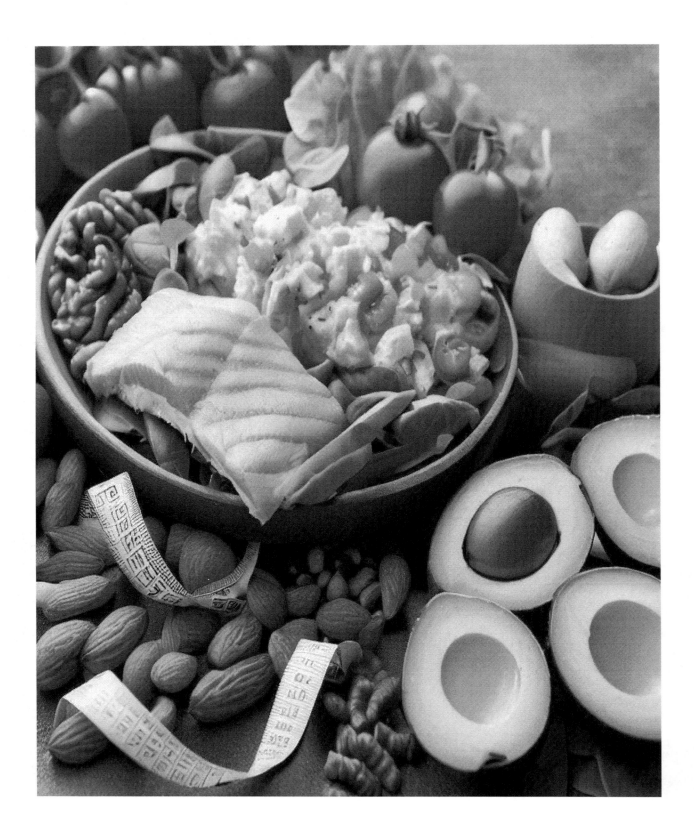

CHAPTER ONE: RECIPES

DELICIOUS BREAKFAST

AVOCADO AND BACON BREAKFAST BOWL

Servings: 2

Prep Time: 10 minutes

Cook Time: 10 minutes

Ingredients:

- 2 avocados, halved and pitted
- 4 strips of bacon, cooked and crumbled
- 4 eggs, fried or poached
- Salt and pepper, to taste
- Chopped fresh chives, for garnish

Instructions:

1. Scoop out a bit of flesh from each avocado half to create a larger well.
2. Place a fried or poached egg into each avocado half.
3. Sprinkle with crumbled bacon, salt, and pepper.
4. Garnish with chopped chives. Enjoy!

Nutritional Information:

Calories: 320 | Protein: 15g | Fat: 25g | Net Carbs: 5g | Fiber: 7g

Benefits: Avocado provides healthy fats and fiber, while eggs and bacon supply protein, making this breakfast both satisfying and nourishing.

Recipe Modification: Swap bacon with turkey bacon for a leaner option.

SPINACH AND MUSHROOM MINI QUICHES

Servings: 6

Prep Time: 15 minutes

Cook Time: 25 minutes

Ingredients:

- 6 eggs
- 1/2 cup spinach, chopped
- 1/2 cup mushrooms, sliced
- 1/4 cup heavy cream
- Salt and pepper, to taste
- Grated Parmesan cheese, for topping

Instructions:

1. Preheat the oven to 350°F (175°C) and grease a muffin tin.
2. Whisk together eggs and heavy cream.
3. Stir in spinach and mushrooms, and season with salt and pepper.
4. Pour mixture into muffin tin, filling each cup about 3/4 full.
5. Sprinkle grated Parmesan cheese on top.
6. Bake for 20-25 minutes, until quiches are set and slightly golden.
7. Let cool slightly before removing from the tin. Enjoy!

Nutritional Information:

Calories: 130 | Protein: 8g | Fat: 10g | Net Carbs: 2g | Fiber: 2g

Benefits: Eggs provide high-quality protein while spinach and mushrooms offer vitamins and minerals. The heavy cream adds richness and healthy fats.

Recipe Modification: Add diced bell peppers or diced cooked sausage for additional flavor.

COCONUT CHIA PUDDING

Servings: 2

Prep Time: 5 minutes (plus overnight chilling)

Cook Time: 0 minutes

Ingredients:

- 1/4 cup chia seeds
- 1 cup unsweetened coconut milk
- 1 teaspoon vanilla extract
- Low-carb sweetener (e.g., stevia or erythritol), to taste
- Unsweetened shredded coconut, for topping

Instructions:

1. In a bowl, mix chia seeds, coconut milk, vanilla extract, and sweetener.
2. Stir well, ensuring the chia seeds are fully submerged.
3. Cover and refrigerate overnight or for at least 4 hours.
4. Before serving, give the pudding a good stir and top with shredded coconut. Enjoy!

Nutritional Information:

Calories: 170 | Protein: 5g | Fat: 12g | Net Carbs: 3g | Fiber: 10g

Benefits: Chia seeds are a rich source of omega-3 fatty acids and fiber, while coconut milk adds creaminess and a touch of tropical flavor.

Recipe Modification: Add a handful of mixed berries for extra flavor and antioxidants.

ALMOND FLOUR PANCAKES

Servings: 2

Prep Time: 10 minutes

Cook Time: 10 minutes

Ingredients:

- 1 cup almond flour
- 2 eggs
- 1/4 cup unsweetened almond milk
- 1 teaspoon baking powder
- Low-carb sweetener, to taste
- Butter or coconut oil, for cooking

Instructions:

1. In a bowl, whisk almond flour, eggs, almond milk, baking powder, and sweetener until smooth.
2. Heat a non-stick skillet over medium heat and grease with butter or coconut oil.
3. Pour 1/4 cup of batter onto the skillet to form pancakes.
4. Cook until bubbles form on the surface, then flip and cook until golden brown.
5. Repeat with the remaining batter.
6. Serve with sugar-free syrup or berries. Enjoy!

Nutritional Information:

Calories: 300 | Protein: 14g | Fat: 25g | Net Carbs: 4g | Fiber: 3g

Benefits: Almond flour is low in carbs and high in healthy fats, making these pancakes a great alternative to traditional ones.

Recipe Modification: Add a pinch of cinnamon or vanilla extract to the batter for extra flavor.

GREEK YOGURT AND BERRY PARFAIT

Servings: 2

Prep Time: 10 minutes

Cook Time: 0 minutes

Ingredients:

- 1 cup full-fat Greek yogurt
- 1/2 cup mixed berries (e.g., blueberries, raspberries)
- 2 tablespoons chopped nuts (e.g., almonds, walnuts)
- Low-carb sweetener, to taste
- Dash of vanilla extract

Instructions:

1. In each serving glass, layer Greek yogurt, berries, and chopped nuts.
2. Sprinkle with sweetener and a dash of vanilla extract.
3. Repeat the layers until the glasses are filled.
4. Chill in the refrigerator for a few minutes before serving.
5. Enjoy!

Nutritional Information:

Calories: 220 | Protein: 15g | Fat: 14g | Net Carbs: 6g | Fiber: 3g

Benefits: Greek yogurt provides protein and probiotics, while berries offer antioxidants and vitamins.

Recipe Modification: Add a drizzle of sugar-free chocolate sauce for an indulgent twist.

SMOKED SALMON AND CREAM CHEESE WRAP

Servings: 2

Prep Time: 10 minutes

Cook Time: 0 minutes

Ingredients:

- 4 oz. smoked salmon
- 4 tablespoons cream cheese
- 2 large lettuce leaves (e.g., Romaine)
- 1/4 red onion, thinly sliced
- Capers, for garnish

Instructions:

1. Lay the lettuce leaves flat and spread 2 tbsp. of cream cheese on each leaf.
2. Place smoked salmon slices on top of the cream cheese.
3. Add sliced red onion and a sprinkle of capers.
4. Roll up the lettuce leaves, securing them with toothpicks if needed.
5. Enjoy as a wrap or slice into bite-sized rolls.

Nutritional Information:

Calories: 230| Protein: 18g| Fat: 15g | Net Carbs: 3g | Fiber: 3g

Benefits: Smoked salmon is rich in omega-3 fatty acids, and cream cheese provides healthy fats.

Recipe Modification: Add fresh dill or lemon zest for extra flavor.

GREEN EGGS AND HAM SCRAMBLE

Servings: 2

Prep Time: 10 minutes

Cook Time: 10 minutes

Ingredients:

- 4 eggs
- 2 tbsp. heavy cream
- 1 cup fresh spinach, chopped
- 1/4 cup diced cooked ham
- Salt and pepper, to taste
- Olive oil or butter, for cooking

Instructions:

1. In a bowl, whisk eggs and heavy cream together.
2. Heat a skillet over medium heat and add a little olive oil or butter.
3. Add chopped spinach and sauté until wilted.
4. Add diced ham and cook for a minute.
5. Pour in the egg mixture and scramble until cooked to your liking.
6. Season with salt and pepper. Enjoy!

Nutritional Information:

Calories: 270 | Protein: 18g | Fat: 20g | Net Carbs: 2g | Fiber: 2g

Benefits: Spinach offers vitamins and minerals, while eggs and ham provide protein and healthy fats.

Recipe Modification: Add sautéed bell peppers or grated cheese for extra flavor and variety.

KETO BREAKFAST BURRITO BOWL

Servings: 2

Prep Time: 15 minutes

Cook Time: 10 minutes

Ingredients:

- 1 cup cauliflower rice
- 4 oz. cooked ground turkey or sausage
- 2 eggs, scrambled
- 1/4 cup shredded cheddar cheese
- 1/4 avocado, sliced
- Salsa or hot sauce, for garnish

Instructions:

1. In a skillet, sauté cauliflower rice until tender.
2. Add cooked ground turkey or sausage and warm through.
3. Push the mixture to one side of the skillet and scramble eggs on the other side.
4. Mix everything together and top with shredded cheese.
5. Serve in a bowl, garnished with avocado and a drizzle of salsa or hot sauce. Enjoy!

Nutritional Information:

Calories: 320 | Protein: 22g | Fat: 22g | Net Carbs: 6g | Fiber: 3g

Benefits: Cauliflower provides a low-carb alternative to rice, while eggs and turkey/sausage supply protein.

Recipe Modification: Add sautéed bell peppers and onions for added flavor and texture.

LOW-CARB BREAKFAST BURRITO

Servings: 2

Prep Time: 15 minutes

Cook Time: 10 minutes

Ingredients:

- 4 large lettuce leaves (e.g., iceberg or Romaine)
- 4 slices cooked bacon
- 2 eggs, fried or scrambled
- 1/4 cup diced tomatoes
- 1/4 cup diced red onion
- Sour cream, for garnish

Instructions:

1. Lay lettuce leaves flat as wraps.
2. Fill each leaf with cooked bacon, scrambled or fried eggs, diced tomatoes, and red onion.
3. Garnish with a dollop of sour cream.
4. Roll up the lettuce wraps and secure with toothpicks if needed.
5. Enjoy your low-carb breakfast burrito!

Nutritional Information:

Calories: 220 | Protein: 14g | Fat: 16g | Net Carbs: 4g | Fiber: 2g

Benefits: Lettuce wraps replace tortillas, while eggs and bacon provide protein and healthy fats.

Recipe Modification: Add sliced avocado or grated cheese for added creaminess.

CINNAMON WALNUT COTTAGE CHEESE BOWL

Servings: 1

Prep Time: 5 minutes

Cook Time: 0 minutes

Ingredients:

- 1/2 cup full-fat cottage cheese
- 2 tbsp. chopped walnuts
- 1/2 tsp ground cinnamon
- Low-carb sweetener (optional), to taste

Instructions:

1. In a bowl, mix cottage cheese and chopped walnuts.
2. Sprinkle ground cinnamon on top and add sweetener if desired.
3. Stir well and enjoy!

Nutritional Information:

Calories: 250 | Protein: 17g | Fat: 19g | Net Carbs: 5g | Fiber: 2g

Benefits: Cottage cheese is a good source of protein, and walnuts provide healthy fats and omega-3 fatty acids.

Recipe Modification: Add a handful of mixed berries for extra flavor and antioxidants.

SATISFYING LUNCH

GRILLED CHICKEN CAESAR SALAD

Servings: 2

Prep Time: 15 minutes

Cook Time: 15 minutes

Ingredients:

- 2 boneless, skinless chicken breasts
- Salt and pepper, to taste
- Romaine lettuce, chopped
- Caesar dressing (sugar-free), to taste
- Grated Parmesan cheese, for topping
- Crispy bacon bits, for garnish

Instructions:

1. Season chicken breasts with salt and pepper and grill until cooked through.
2. Slice grilled chicken into thin strips.
3. Toss chopped lettuce with Caesar dressing.
4. Top with sliced chicken, grated Parmesan, and bacon bits. Enjoy!

Nutritional Information:

Calories: 350 | Protein: 30g | Fat: 20g | Net Carbs: 6g | Fiber: 3g

Benefits: Chicken offers lean protein, while romaine lettuce provides vitamins and fiber.

Recipe Modification: Add avocado slices for extra creaminess and healthy fats.

TURKEY AVOCADO LETTUCE WRAPS

Servings: 2

Prep Time: 15 minutes

Cook Time: 0 minutes

Ingredients:

- 8 large lettuce leaves (e.g., Bibb or iceberg)
- 8 oz. sliced deli turkey
- 1 avocado, sliced
- 1/2 cup diced tomatoes
- Mustard or mayo (sugar-free), for dressing

Instructions:

1. Lay lettuce leaves flat as wraps.
2. Layer turkey slices, avocado, and diced tomatoes on each leaf.
3. Drizzle with mustard or mayo.
4. Roll up the lettuce wraps and secure with toothpicks if needed.
5. Enjoy your turkey avocado wraps!

Nutritional Information:

Calories: 280 | Protein: 20g | Fat: 18g | Net Carbs: 6g | Fiber: 4g

Benefits: Turkey offers protein, while avocado provides healthy fats and fiber.

Recipe Modification: Add sliced cucumber or red onion for extra crunch and flavor.

ZUCCHINI NOODLES WITH PESTO AND CHERRY TOMATOES

Servings: 2

Prep Time: 15 minutes

Cook Time: 5 minutes

Ingredients:

- 2 medium zucchinis, spiralized
- 1/4 cup pesto sauce (sugar-free)
- 1 cup cherry tomatoes, halved
- Grated Parmesan cheese, for topping

Instructions:

1. Heat a pan over medium heat and add spiralized zucchini.
2. Cook for a few minutes until slightly softened.
3. Toss zucchini noodles with pesto sauce.
4. Top with halved cherry tomatoes and grated Parmesan.
5. Enjoy your zucchini noodle bowl!

Nutritional Information:

Calories: 250 | Protein: 8g | Fat: 20g | Net Carbs: 6g | Fiber: 4g

Benefits: Zucchini offers a low-carb pasta alternative, and pesto provides healthy fats from nuts and olive oil.

Recipe Modification: Add grilled chicken or shrimp for extra protein.

TUNA SALAD LETTUCE WRAPS

Servings: 2

Prep Time: 10 minutes

Cook Time: 0 minutes

Ingredients:

- 1 can (5 oz.) tuna, drained
- 2 tbsp. mayonnaise (sugar-free)
- 1/4 cup diced celery
- 1/4 cup diced red onion
- Lettuce leaves for wrapping
- Sliced cucumber, for serving

Instructions:

1. In a bowl, mix tuna, mayonnaise, celery, and red onion.
2. Lay lettuce leaves flat as wraps.
3. Spoon tuna salad onto each leaf.
4. Roll up the lettuce wraps and serve with sliced cucumber.
5. Enjoy your tuna salad wraps!

Nutritional Information:

Calories: 220 | Protein: 20g | Fat: 15g | Net Carbs: 3g | Fiber: 2g

Benefits: Tuna offers protein, and celery adds crunch and fiber.

Recipe Modification: Add chopped pickles or chopped hard-boiled eggs for extra flavor and texture.

BROCCOLI AND CHEDDAR STUFFED CHICKEN

Servings: 2

Prep Time: 15 minutes

Cook Time: 25 minutes

Ingredients:

- 2 boneless, skinless chicken breasts
- Salt and pepper, to taste
- 1 cup steamed broccoli florets
- 1/2 cup shredded cheddar cheese
- Paprika, for sprinkling

Instructions:

1. Preheat the oven to 375°F (190°C).
2. Season chicken breasts with salt and pepper.
3. Cut a slit in each chicken breast to create a pocket.
4. Stuff each pocket with steamed broccoli and cheddar cheese.
5. Sprinkle paprika on top.
6. Bake in the preheated oven for 20-25 minutes or until chicken is cooked through.
7. Enjoy your cheesy stuffed chicken!

Nutritional Information:

Calories: 350 | Protein: 40g | Fat: 16g | Net Carbs: 5g | Fiber: 2g

Benefits: Chicken offers lean protein, while broccoli provides fiber and vitamins.

Recipe Modification: Add diced ham or sautéed mushrooms to the stuffing for added flavor.

CAULIFLOWER FRIED RICE

Servings: 2

Prep Time: 15 minutes

Cook Time: 10 minutes

Ingredients:

- 2 cups cauliflower rice
- 8 oz. cooked shrimp or diced chicken
- 1/2 cup diced mixed vegetables (e.g., bell peppers, carrots)
- 2 eggs, scrambled
- 2 tbsps. soy sauce (low-sodium)
- Sesame oil, for cooking

Instructions:

1. In a pan, heat a bit of sesame oil and sauté diced vegetables until slightly tender.
2. Push vegetables to one side of the pan and scramble eggs on the other side.
3. Add cooked shrimp or chicken and cauliflower rice to the pan.
4. Drizzle with soy sauce and stir-fry until heated through.
5. Enjoy your flavorful cauliflower fried rice!

Nutritional Information:

Calories: 320 | Protein: 30g | Fat: 12g | Net Carbs: 10g | Fiber: 2g

Benefits: Cauliflower rice is low-carb, and shrimp/chicken provides protein.

Recipe Modification: Add chopped scallions and ginger for an extra kick of flavor.

EGG SALAD LETTUCE WRAPS

Servings: 2

Prep Time: 10 minutes

Cook Time: 10 minutes (for hard-boiled eggs)

Ingredients:

- 4 hard-boiled eggs, peeled and chopped
- 2 tbsps. mayonnaise (sugar-free)
- 1 teaspoon Dijon mustard
- Salt and pepper, to taste
- Lettuce leaves for wrapping

Instructions:

1. In a bowl, mix chopped hard-boiled eggs, mayonnaise, Dijon mustard, salt, and pepper.
2. Lay lettuce leaves flat as wraps.
3. Spoon egg salad onto each leaf.
4. Roll up the lettuce wraps.
5. Enjoy your egg salad wraps!

Nutritional Information:

Calories: 280 | Protein: 15g | Fat: 22g | Net Carbs: 2g | Fiber: 3g

Benefits: Eggs offer protein, while mayo and mustard add flavor.

Recipe Modification: Add chopped celery or pickles for extra crunch.

BEEF AND BROCCOLI STIR-FRY

Servings: 2

Prep Time: 15 minutes

Cook Time: 15 minutes

Ingredients:

- 8 oz. sliced beef (e.g., flank steak)
- Salt and pepper, to taste
- 1 cup broccoli florets
- 2 tbsps. soy sauce (low-sodium)
- 1 teaspoon sesame oil
- Garlic powder, to taste

Instructions:

1. Season sliced beef with salt and pepper.
2. In a pan, heat sesame oil and stir-fry beef until browned.
3. Add broccoli florets and stir-fry until tender-crisp.
4. Drizzle with soy sauce and sprinkle with garlic powder.
5. Enjoy your quick and tasty beef and broccoli stir-fry!

Nutritional Information:

Calories: 300 | Protein: 25g | Fat: 18g | Net Carbs: 5g | Fiber: 2g

Benefits: Beef provides protein and iron, while broccoli offers fiber and vitamins.

Recipe Modification: Add sliced bell peppers or mushrooms for additional veggies.

CREAMY AVOCADO TUNA SALAD

Servings: 2

Prep Time: 10 minutes

Cook Time: 0 minutes

Ingredients:

- 1 can (5 oz.) tuna, drained
- 1 ripe avocado, mashed
- 2 tbsps. Greek yogurt
- 1/4 cup diced red onion
- Salt and pepper, to taste

Instructions:

1. In a bowl, mix drained tuna, mashed avocado, Greek yogurt, diced red onion, salt, and pepper.
2. Serve on its own or with cucumber slices.
3. Enjoy your creamy avocado tuna salad!

Nutritional Information:

Calories: 290 | Protein: 20g | Fat: 20g | Net Carbs: 6g | Fiber: 6g

Benefits: Tuna offers protein, and avocado provides healthy fats and fiber.

Recipe Modification: Add chopped cilantro or lime juice for a burst of flavor.

MEDITERRANEAN CHICKEN SALAD

Servings: 2

Prep Time: 20 minutes

Cook Time: 15 minutes

Ingredients:

- 2 boneless, skinless chicken breasts
- Salt and pepper, to taste
- Mixed salad greens
- Cherry tomatoes, halved
- Cucumber, sliced
- Red onion, thinly sliced
- Kalamata olives
- Feta cheese, crumbled
- Balsamic vinaigrette (sugar-free)

Instructions:

1. Season chicken breasts with salt and pepper and grill until cooked through.
2. Slice grilled chicken into thin strips.
3. Toss salad greens with cherry tomatoes, cucumber, red onion, olives, and feta cheese.
4. Top with sliced chicken.
5. Drizzle with balsamic vinaigrette.
6. Enjoy your Mediterranean-inspired chicken salad!

Nutritional Information:

Calories: 320 | Protein: 30g | Fat: 18g | Net Carbs: 7g | Fiber: 4g

Benefits: Chicken offers lean protein, while olives and feta cheese add Mediterranean flair.

Recipe Modification: Add roasted red peppers or artichoke hearts for extra depth of flavor.

NUTRIENT-PACKED DINNER

BAKED SALMON WITH ASPARAGUS AND LEMON

Servings: 2

Prep Time: 10 minutes

Cook Time: 20 minutes

Ingredients:

- 2 salmon fillets
- Salt and pepper, to taste
- 1 bunch asparagus, trimmed
- 1 lemon, sliced
- Olive oil
- Fresh dill, for garnish

Instructions:

1. Preheat the oven to 375°F (190°C).
2. Season salmon fillets with salt and pepper.
3. Place salmon and asparagus on a baking sheet.
4. Drizzle with olive oil and top with lemon slices.
5. Bake for about 15-20 minutes, until salmon flakes easily.
6. Garnish with fresh dill.
7. Enjoy your nutritious baked salmon!

Nutritional Information:

Calories: 350 | Protein: 30g | Fat: 22g | Net Carbs: 4g | Fiber: 2g

Benefits: Salmon is rich in omega-3 fatty acids, and asparagus provides vitamins and fiber.

Recipe Modification: Add minced garlic to the olive oil for extra flavor.

GRILLED STEAK WITH ROASTED BRUSSELS SPROUTS

Servings: 2

Prep Time: 15 minutes

Cook Time: 25 minutes

Ingredients:

- 2 ribeye steaks
- Salt and pepper, to taste
- 1 lb. Brussels sprouts, halved
- Olive oil
- Balsamic vinegar (sugar-free), for drizzling

Instructions:

1. Preheat the grill.
2. Season steaks with salt and pepper and grill to desired doneness.
3. Toss halved Brussels sprouts with olive oil, salt, and pepper.
4. Roast Brussels sprouts in the oven at 400°F (200°C) for about 20 minutes.
5. Drizzle with balsamic vinegar before serving.
6. Enjoy your hearty grilled steak and Brussels sprouts!

Nutritional Information:

Calories: 450 | Protein: 40g | Fat: 28g | Net Carbs: 9g | Fiber: 4g

Benefits: Steak provides protein and iron, while Brussels sprouts offer vitamins and fiber.

Recipe Modification: Add crumbled blue cheese on top of the Brussels sprouts for a tangy twist.

STUFFED BELL PEPPERS WITH GROUND TURKEY

Servings: 2

Prep Time: 15 minutes

Cook Time: 30 minutes

Ingredients:

- 2 large bell peppers, halved and seeds removed
- 8 oz. ground turkey
- 1/2 cup cauliflower rice
- 1/4 cup diced tomatoes
- 1/4 cup shredded cheddar cheese
- Olive oil
- Salt and pepper, to taste

Instructions:

1. Preheat the oven to 375°F (190°C).
2. In a skillet, cook ground turkey until browned.
3. Add cauliflower rice and diced tomatoes to the skillet, and season with salt and pepper.
4. Spoon turkey mixture into bell pepper halves.
5. Top with shredded cheddar cheese.
6. Bake for about 20-25 minutes, until peppers are tender.
7. Enjoy your flavorful stuffed bell peppers!

Nutritional Information:

Calories: 320 | Protein: 25g | Fat: 20g | Net Carbs: 9g | Fiber: 3g

Benefits: Ground turkey provides protein, and bell peppers are rich in vitamins.

Recipe Modification: Add diced zucchini or spinach to the turkey mixture for added veggies.

GARLIC BUTTER SHRIMP AND ZOODLES

Servings: 2

Prep Time: 15 minutes

Cook Time: 10 minutes

Ingredients:

- 8 oz. shrimp, peeled and deveined
- Salt and pepper, to taste
- 2 medium zucchinis, spiralized
- 2 tbsps. unsalted butter
- 2 cloves garlic, minced
- Lemon zest, for garnish

Instructions:

1. Season shrimp with salt and pepper.
2. In a pan, melt butter and sauté minced garlic until fragrant.
3. Add shrimp and cook until pink and opaque.
4. Push shrimp to one side of the pan and add spiralized zucchini.
5. Toss zoodles in garlic butter and warm through.
6. Serve shrimp and zoodles together, garnished with lemon zest.
7. Enjoy your garlic butter shrimp and zoodles!

Nutritional Information:

Calories: 300 | Protein: 25g | Fat: 20g | Net Carbs: 7g | Fiber: 3g

Benefits: Shrimp offers protein, while zoodles are a low-carb pasta alternative.

Recipe Modification: Add crushed red pepper flakes for a touch of heat.

BAKED STUFFED PORTOBELLO MUSHROOMS

Servings: 2

Prep Time: 15 minutes

Cook Time: 20 minutes

Ingredients:

- 4 large Portobello mushrooms, stems removed
- 1/2 lb. ground beef or turkey
- 1/4 cup diced bell peppers
- 1/4 cup diced onion
- 1/4 cup marinara sauce (sugar-free)
- 1/4 cup shredded mozzarella cheese
- Olive oil
- Italian seasoning, to taste

Instructions:

1. Preheat the oven to 375°F (190°C).
2. Place Portobello mushrooms on a baking sheet.
3. In a skillet, cook ground beef or turkey until browned.
4. Add diced bell peppers and onions to the skillet and sauté.
5. Stir in marinara sauce and Italian seasoning.
6. Spoon the meat mixture into the mushroom caps.
7. Top with shredded mozzarella cheese.
8. Bake for about 15-20 minutes, until cheese is melted and mushrooms are tender.
9. Enjoy your savory stuffed Portobello mushrooms!

Nutritional Information:

Calories: 350 | Protein: 25g | Fat: 22g | Net Carbs: 9g | Fiber: 2g

Benefits: Ground beef or turkey provides protein, and Portobello mushrooms offer vitamins.

Recipe Modification: Add diced tomatoes or chopped spinach to the meat mixture.

CAULIFLOWER CRUST PIZZA

Servings: 2

Prep Time: 15 minutes

Cook Time: 20 minutes

Ingredients:

- 1 cauliflower crust (store-bought or homemade)
- 1/4 cup sugar-free pizza sauce
- 1 cup shredded mozzarella cheese
- Toppings of your choice (e.g., pepperoni, bell peppers, mushrooms)

Instructions:

1. Preheat the oven according to cauliflower crust package instructions.
2. Spread pizza sauce over the crust.
3. Sprinkle shredded mozzarella cheese on top.
4. Add your favorite toppings.
5. Bake the pizza according to crust package instructions.
6. Enjoy your delicious low-carb cauliflower crust pizza!

Nutritional Information:

Calories: 300 | Protein: 20g | Fat: 18g | Net Carbs: 8g | Fiber: 3g

Benefits: Cauliflower crust replaces traditional high-carb pizza crust.

Recipe Modification: Use a variety of colorful vegetables for extra nutrients.

LEMON HERB GRILLED CHICKEN WITH STEAMED BROCCOLI

Servings: 2

Prep Time: 15 minutes

Cook Time: 20 minutes

Ingredients:

- 2 boneless, skinless chicken breasts
- Salt and pepper, to taste
- Zest and juice of 1 lemon
- 1 tsp dried herbs (e.g., thyme, rosemary)
- 1 lb. broccoli florets
- Olive oil

Instructions:

1. Preheat the grill.
2. Season chicken breasts with salt, pepper, lemon zest, and dried herbs.
3. Grill chicken until cooked through.
4. Steam broccoli until tender.
5. Drizzle broccoli with olive oil and lemon juice.
6. Serve chicken with steamed broccoli.
7. Enjoy your lemon herb grilled chicken with a side of veggies!

Nutritional Information:

Calories: 320 | Protein: 30g | Fat: 18g | Net Carbs: 8g | Fiber: 4g

Benefits: Chicken offers lean protein, and broccoli provides vitamins and fiber.

Recipe Modification: Add minced garlic to the chicken marinade for extra flavor.

SPINACH AND FETA STUFFED CHICKEN BREAST

Servings: 2

Prep Time: 15 minutes

Cook Time: 25 minutes

Ingredients:

- 2 boneless, skinless chicken breasts
- Salt and pepper, to taste
- 1 cup fresh spinach, chopped
- 1/4 cup crumbled feta cheese
- Olive oil
- Garlic powder, to taste

Instructions:

1. Preheat the oven to 375°F (190°C).
2. Season chicken breasts with salt and pepper.
3. In a bowl, mix chopped spinach and crumbled feta.
4. Cut a slit in each chicken breast to create a pocket.
5. Stuff each pocket with the spinach and feta mixture.
6. Drizzle with olive oil and sprinkle with garlic powder.
7. Bake for about 20-25 minutes, until chicken is cooked through.
8. Enjoy your flavorful spinach and feta stuffed chicken!

Nutritional Information:

Calories: 320 | Protein: 30g | Fat: 18g | Net Carbs: 4g | Fiber: 1g

Benefits: Chicken offers protein, while spinach and feta provide vitamins and flavor.

Recipe Modification: Add sun-dried tomatoes or olives to the stuffing for extra depth.

EGGPLANT PARMESAN

Servings: 2

Prep Time: 20 minutes

Cook Time: 30 minutes

Ingredients:

- 1 medium eggplant, sliced
- Salt, to taste
- 1/2 cup almond flour
- 2 eggs, beaten
- 1 cup sugar-free marinara sauce
- 1 cup shredded mozzarella cheese
- Olive oil

Instructions:

1. Preheat the oven to 375°F (190°C).
2. Lay eggplant slices on paper towels and sprinkle with salt to draw out moisture.
3. Dip eggplant slices in beaten eggs, then coat with almond flour.
4. In a pan, heat olive oil and sauté eggplant until golden brown on both sides.
5. Layer eggplant slices in a baking dish, then top with marinara sauce and mozzarella cheese.
6. Bake for about 15-20 minutes, until cheese is melted and bubbly.
7. Enjoy your flavorful eggplant Parmesan!

Nutritional Information:

Calories: 340 | Protein: 20g | Fat: 24g | Net Carbs: 10g | Fiber: 5g

Benefits: Eggplant provides vitamins and fiber, while almond flour adds a crispy coating.

Recipe Modification: Add chopped fresh basil on top before baking for extra freshness.

BEEF STIR-FRY WITH BROCCOLI AND PEPPERS

Servings: 2

Prep Time: 15 minutes

Cook Time: 15 minutes

Ingredients:

- 8 oz. sliced beef (e.g., sirloin or flank steak)
- Salt and pepper, to taste
- 1 cup broccoli florets
- 1 bell pepper, sliced
- 2 tbsps. soy sauce (low-sodium)
- 1 teaspoon sesame oil

Instructions:

1. Season sliced beef with salt and pepper.
2. In a pan, heat sesame oil and stir-fry beef until browned.
3. Add broccoli florets and sliced bell pepper.
4. Drizzle with soy sauce and stir-fry until veggies are tender-crisp.
5. Enjoy your quick and flavorful beef stir-fry!

Nutritional Information:

Calories: 330 | Protein: 25g | Fat: 22g | Net Carbs: 6g | Fiber: 2g

Benefits: Beef provides protein and iron, while broccoli and bell pepper add vitamins and color.

Recipe Modification: Add sliced mushrooms or chopped green beans for extra veggies.

WHOLESOME SNACK AND APPETIZER

GUACAMOLE AND VEGGIE STICKS

Servings: 2

Prep Time: 10 minutes

Ingredients:

- 2 ripe avocados, mashed
- 1/4 cup diced tomatoes
- 2 tbsps. diced red onion
- 1 clove garlic, minced
- Lime juice, to taste
- Salt and pepper, to taste
- Assorted veggie sticks (e.g., cucumber, bell pepper)

Instructions:

1. In a bowl, combine mashed avocados, diced tomatoes, red onion, minced garlic, lime juice, salt, and pepper.
2. Serve with assorted veggie sticks.
3. Enjoy your creamy guacamole and crunchy veggies!

Nutritional Information:

Calories: 200 | Protein: 3g | Fat: 18g | Net Carbs: 8g | Fiber: 6g

Benefits: Avocados provide healthy fats, and veggies add vitamins and fiber.

Recipe Modification: Add chopped cilantro and a touch of cayenne pepper for extra flavor.

DEVILED EGGS

Servings: 2

Prep Time: 15 minutes

Ingredients:

- 4 hard-boiled eggs, peeled and halved
- 2 tbsps. mayonnaise (sugar-free)
- 1 tsp Dijon mustard
- Salt and pepper, to taste
- Paprika, for garnish

Instructions:

1. In a bowl, mix egg yolks, mayonnaise, Dijon mustard, salt, and pepper.
2. Spoon or pipe the mixture into the egg white halves.
3. Sprinkle with paprika.
4. Enjoy your classic deviled eggs!

Nutritional Information:

Calories: 160 | Protein: 10g | Fat: 12g | Net Carbs: 1g | Fiber: 0g

Benefits: Eggs offer protein and healthy fats.

Recipe Modification: Add a dash of hot sauce or minced herbs to the filling.

CUCUMBER AND CREAM CHEESE BITES

Servings: 2

Prep Time: 10 minutes

Ingredients:

- 1 cucumber, sliced
- 2 oz. cream cheese
- Smoked salmon or deli meat (optional)
- Fresh dill or chives, for garnish

Instructions:

1. Spread a thin layer of cream cheese on each cucumber slice.
2. Top with smoked salmon or deli meat if desired.
3. Garnish with fresh dill or chives.
4. Enjoy your refreshing cucumber and cream cheese bites!

Nutritional Information:

Calories: 150 | Protein: 5g | Fat: 12g | Net Carbs: 3g | Fiber: 1g

Benefits: Cucumbers provide hydration, and cream cheese adds creaminess.

Recipe Modification: Add a slice of avocado for extra texture.

ALMOND-STUFFED DATES WRAPPED IN BACON

Servings: 2

Prep Time: 15 minutes

Cook Time: 15 minutes

Ingredients:

- 6 Medjool dates, pitted
- 12 whole almonds
- 6 slices bacon, halved

Instructions:

1. Preheat the oven to 375°F (190°C).
2. Stuff each date with 2 almonds.
3. Wrap each stuffed date with a half slice of bacon and secure with a toothpick.
4. Place wrapped dates on a baking sheet.
5. Bake for about 10-15 minutes, until bacon is crispy.
6. Enjoy your sweet and savory bacon-wrapped treats!

Nutritional Information:

Calories: 200 | Protein: 4g | Fat: 10g | Net Carbs: 20g | Fiber: 3g

Benefits: Dates provide natural sweetness, and almonds offer protein and healthy fats.

Recipe Modification: Use turkey bacon for a leaner option.

SMOKED SALMON CUCUMBER BITES

Servings: 2

Prep Time: 10 minutes

Ingredients:

- 1 cucumber, sliced
- 2 oz. cream cheese
- Smoked salmon slices
- Fresh dill, for garnish

Instructions:

1. Spread a thin layer of cream cheese on each cucumber slice.
2. Top with a slice of smoked salmon.
3. Garnish with fresh dill.
4. Enjoy your elegant smoked salmon cucumber bites!

Nutritional Information:

Calories: 180 | Protein: 10g | Fat: 12g | Net Carbs: 3g | Fiber: 1g

Benefits: Smoked salmon offers protein and omega-3 fatty acids.

Recipe Modification: Add a caper or a sprinkle of lemon zest for extra flavor.

SPICY BUFFALO CAULIFLOWER BITES

Servings: 2

Prep Time: 15 minutes

Cook Time: 25 minutes

Ingredients:

- 2 cups cauliflower florets
- 2 tbsps. olive oil
- Salt and pepper, to taste
- 1/4 cup hot sauce (sugar-free)
- 2 tbsps. melted butter
- Ranch or blue cheese dressing, for dipping

Instructions:

1. Preheat the oven to 425°F (220°C).
2. Toss cauliflower florets with olive oil, salt, and pepper.
3. Spread cauliflower on a baking sheet and roast for about 20 minutes, until golden.
4. In a bowl, mix hot sauce and melted butter.
5. Toss roasted cauliflower in the hot sauce mixture.
6. Serve with ranch or blue cheese dressing.
7. Enjoy your spicy buffalo cauliflower bites!

Nutritional Information:

Calories: 180 | Protein: 4g | Fat: 14g | Net Carbs: 5g | Fiber: 2g

Benefits: Cauliflower provides vitamins, and hot sauce adds a kick of flavor.

Recipe Modification: Add a pinch of garlic powder for extra depth.

ZUCCHINI PARMESAN CRISPS

Servings: 2

Prep Time: 15 minutes

Cook Time: 15 minutes

Ingredients:

- 1 medium zucchini, sliced
- 1/4 cup almond flour
- 1/4 cup grated Parmesan cheese
- 1 teaspoon Italian seasoning
- Salt and pepper, to taste
- 1 egg, beaten

Instructions:

1. Preheat the oven to 425°F (220°C).
2. In a bowl, mix almond flour, grated Parmesan, Italian seasoning, salt, and pepper.
3. Dip zucchini slices in beaten egg, then coat with the almond flour mixture.
4. Place coated zucchini slices on a baking sheet.
5. Bake for about 10-15 minutes, until crispy.
6. Enjoy your crunchy zucchini Parmesan crisps!

Nutritional Information:

Calories: 150 | Protein: 8g | Fat: 10g | Net Carbs: 6g | Fiber: 2g

Benefits: Zucchini provides vitamins, and Parmesan cheese adds savory flavor.

Recipe Modification: Add a pinch of red pepper flakes for a bit of heat.

CAPRESE SKEWERS

Servings: 2

Prep Time: 15 minutes

Ingredients:

- Cherry tomatoes
- Fresh mozzarella balls
- Fresh basil leaves
- Balsamic vinegar (sugar-free), for drizzling
- Olive oil
- Salt and pepper, to taste

Instructions:

1. Thread cherry tomatoes, mozzarella balls, and basil leaves onto small skewers.
2. Drizzle with balsamic vinegar and olive oil.
3. Season with salt and pepper.
4. Enjoy your delightful Caprese skewers!

Nutritional Information:

Calories: 150 | Protein: 10g | Fat: 12g | Net Carbs: 4g | Fiber: 1g

Benefits: Tomatoes offer vitamins, and mozzarella adds protein and creaminess.

Recipe Modification: Use a sprinkle of dried basil if fresh is not available.

MIXED NUTS AND CHEESE PLATTER

Servings: 2

Prep Time: 10 minutes

Ingredients:

- Assorted mixed nuts (e.g., almonds, walnuts, pecans)
- Assorted cheese slices (e.g., cheddar, Swiss)
- Olives and pickles
- Berries or sliced veggies (for garnish)

Instructions:

1. Arrange mixed nuts and cheese slices on a platter.
2. Add olives, pickles, and berries or veggies for variety.
3. Enjoy your satisfying mixed nuts and cheese platter!

Nutritional Information:

Calories: 250 | Protein: 10g | Fat: 20g | Net Carbs: 5g | Fiber: 3g

Benefits: Nuts provide healthy fats, and cheese offers protein.

Recipe Modification: Add a sprinkle of dried herbs on the cheese for extra flavor.

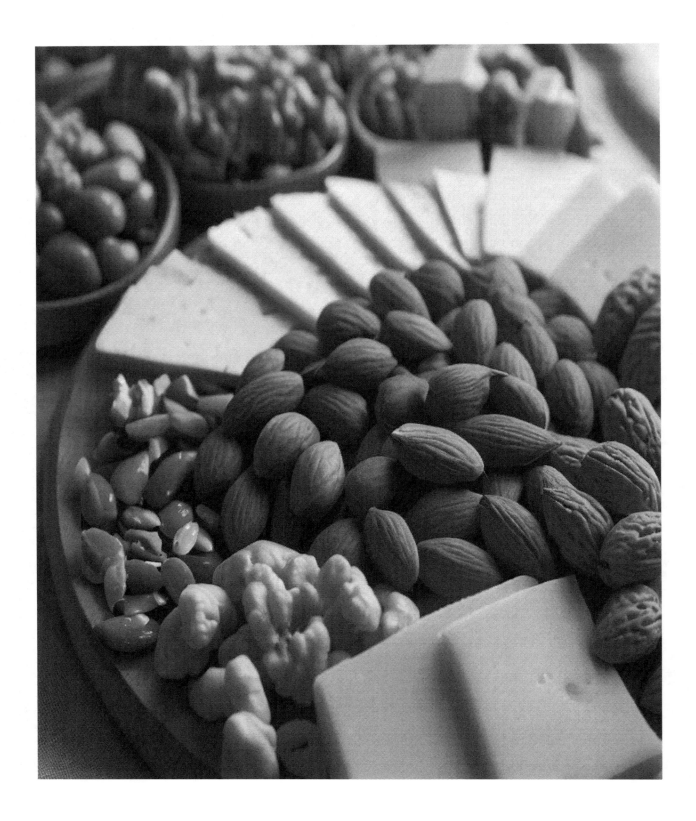

SOUPS AND SALADS

MEXICAN CAULIFLOWER RICE SALAD

Servings: 4-6

Prep Time: 15 minutes

Ingredients:

4 cups cauliflower rice (fresh or frozen)

- 1 can black beans, drained and rinsed
- 1 cup diced bell peppers
- 1/2 cup diced red onion
- 1/4 cup chopped fresh cilantro
- Juice of 1 lime
- 2 tablespoons olive oil
- 1 teaspoon cumin
- 1 teaspoon chili powder
- Salt and pepper to taste

Instructions:

1. In a bowl, mix cauliflower rice, black beans, diced bell peppers, and diced red onion, chopped cilantro, lime juice, olive oil, cumin, chili powder, salt, and pepper.
2. Toss gently to combine.
3. Serve as a flavorful and low-carb salad.

Nutritional Information:

Calories: 200 (per serving) | Protein: 8g | Fat: 10g | Net Carbs: 7g | Fiber: 3g

Key Benefits: Cauliflower rice offers a low-carb base, while black beans provide protein and fiber.

Recipe Modification: Top with diced avocado or a dollop of Greek yogurt.

ZUCCHINI AND TOMATO SALAD

Servings: 2-3

Prep Time: 10 minutes

Cook Time: 0 minutes

Ingredients:

- 2 medium zucchinis, sliced
- 1 cup cherry tomatoes, halved
- 1/4 cup chopped red onion
- 2 tablespoons olive oil
- 1 tablespoon balsamic vinegar
- 1 tablespoon chopped fresh basil
- Salt and pepper to taste

Instructions:

1. In a bowl, combine sliced zucchinis, halved cherry tomatoes, and chopped red onion.
2. Drizzle olive oil and balsamic vinegar over the mixture.
3. Add chopped fresh basil, salt, and pepper. Toss to combine.
4. Serve zucchini and tomato salad as a refreshing and light side.

Nutritional Information:

Calories: 100 (per serving) | Protein: 2g | Fat: 8g | Net Carbs: 5g | Fiber: 2g

Key Benefits: Zucchini offers vitamins and minerals, while tomatoes add antioxidants.

Recipe Modification: Add crumbled feta cheese for a tangy twist.

TOMATO BASIL SOUP WITH PARMESAN CRISPS

Servings: 4-6

Prep Time: 10 minutes

Cook Time: 25 minutes

Ingredients:

- 4 cups diced tomatoes (canned or fresh)
- 2 cups chicken or vegetable broth
- 1/2 cup heavy cream
- 1/4 cup chopped fresh basil
- 2 cloves garlic, minced
- 1 small onion, diced
- 2 tablespoons olive oil
- Salt and pepper to taste
- Grated Parmesan cheese for garnish

Instructions:

1. In a pot, heat olive oil and sauté diced onion and minced garlic until translucent.
2. Add diced tomatoes and cook for a few minutes.
3. Pour in chicken or vegetable broth and bring to a simmer.
4. Let the soup simmer for about 15-20 minutes.
5. Use an immersion blender to puree the soup until smooth.
6. Stir in heavy cream and chopped fresh basil.
7. Season with salt and pepper.
8. Serve hot, garnished with grated Parmesan cheese.

Nutritional Information:

Calories: 250 (per serving) | Protein: 5g | Fat: 20g | Net Carbs: 9g | Fiber: 2g

Key Benefits: Tomatoes provide vitamins and antioxidants, while basil adds fresh flavor.

Recipe Modification: Serve with homemade Parmesan crisps for added crunch.

ASIAN CABBAGE SALAD WITH GRILLED STEAK

Servings: 2-3

Prep Time: 20 minutes

Cook Time: 10 minutes

Ingredients:

- 1 pound steak (such as flank or sirloin)
- 6 cups shredded cabbage
- 1 cup shredded carrots
- 1/4 cup sliced green onions
- 1/4 cup chopped fresh cilantro
- 2 tablespoons sesame oil
- 2 tablespoons soy sauce (or tamari for gluten-free)
- 1 tablespoon rice vinegar
- 1 teaspoon grated fresh ginger
- Salt and pepper to taste

Instructions:

1. Preheat a grill or grill pan.
2. Season steak with salt and pepper.
3. Grill steak for about 4-5 minutes per side for medium-rare, or until desired doneness.
4. Let the steak rest before slicing.
5. In a large bowl, combine shredded cabbage, shredded carrots, sliced green onions, and chopped cilantro.
6. In a small bowl, whisk together sesame oil, soy sauce, rice vinegar, grated fresh ginger, salt, and pepper to make the dressing.
7. Add sliced grilled steak on top of the salad.
8. Drizzle the dressing over the salad.
9. Toss gently to coat.
10. Serve as an Asian-inspired and satisfying salad.

Nutritional Information:

Calories: 350 (per serving) | Protein: 30g | Fat: 20g | Net Carbs: 9g | Fiber: 4g

Key Benefits: Grilled steak provides protein, while cabbage and carrots offer vitamins and fiber.

Recipe Modification: Top with toasted sesame seeds for added crunch.

SPICY CHICKEN AND KALE SOUP

Servings: 4-6

Prep Time: 15 minutes

Cook Time: 30 minutes

Ingredients:

- 2 boneless, skinless chicken breasts, diced
- 4 cups chicken broth
- 2 cups chopped kale
- 1 can diced tomatoes
- 1 small onion, diced
- 2 cloves garlic, minced
- 1 teaspoon cumin
- 1 teaspoon chili powder
- 1/2 teaspoon cayenne pepper (adjust to taste)
- Salt and pepper to taste
- Olive oil for cooking

Instructions:

1. In a pot, heat olive oil and sauté diced onion and minced garlic until translucent.
2. Add diced chicken and cook until no longer pink.
3. Stir in cumin, chili powder, cayenne pepper, salt, and pepper.

4. Pour in chicken broth and bring to a boil.
5. Add chopped kale and diced tomatoes, then reduce to a simmer.
6. Let the soup simmer until the kale is tender.
7. Adjust seasoning to taste.
8. Serve hot.

Nutritional Information:

Calories: 250 (per serving) | Protein: 20g | Fat: 10g | Net Carbs: 8g | Fiber: 3g

Key Benefits: Chicken provides protein, while kale offers vitamins and antioxidants.

Recipe Modification: Top with a dollop of sour cream for extra creaminess.

GRILLED SHRIMP SALAD WITH LEMON HERB DRESSING

Servings: 2-3

Prep Time: 15 minutes

Cook Time: 10 minutes

Ingredients:

- 1 pound large shrimp, peeled and deveined
- 6 cups mixed salad greens
- 1 cup cherry tomatoes, halved
- 1/4 cup sliced red onion
- 1/4 cup crumbled feta cheese
- 2 tablespoons chopped fresh parsley
- Juice of 1 lemon
- 2 tablespoons olive oil
- 1 teaspoon Dijon mustard
- Salt and pepper to taste

Instructions:

1. Preheat a grill or grill pan.
2. Season shrimp with salt and pepper.
3. Grill shrimp for about 2-3 minutes per side or until cooked through.
4. In a bowl, whisk together lemon juice, olive oil, Dijon mustard, salt, and pepper to make the dressing.
5. In a large salad bowl, combine mixed salad greens, halved cherry tomatoes, sliced red onion, crumbled feta cheese, and chopped parsley.
6. Add grilled shrimp on top.
7. Drizzle the lemon herb dressing over the salad.
8. Toss gently to coat.
9. Serve as a satisfying and light salad.

Nutritional Information:

Calories: 300 (per serving) | Protein: 25g | Fat: 15g | Net Carbs: 9g | Fiber: 3g

Key Benefits: Shrimp offers protein and omega-3 fatty acids, while mixed greens provide vitamins and minerals.

Recipe Modification: Add sliced avocado for extra creaminess.

CAULIFLOWER AND LEEK SOUP

Servings: 4-6

Prep Time: 15 minutes

Cook Time: 25 minutes

Ingredients:

- 1 medium cauliflower head, chopped
- 2 leeks, white and light green parts, sliced
- 4 cups chicken or vegetable broth
- 1 cup heavy cream
- 2 tablespoons butter
- Salt and pepper to taste
- Chopped fresh chives for garnish

Instructions:

1. In a pot, melt butter and sauté sliced leeks until tender.
2. Add chopped cauliflower and cook for a few minutes.
3. Pour in chicken or vegetable broth and bring to a simmer.
4. Let the soup simmer until the cauliflower is tender.
5. Use an immersion blender to puree the soup until smooth.
6. Stir in heavy cream and season with salt and pepper.
7. Serve hot, garnished with chopped chives.

Nutritional Information:

Calories: 250 (per serving) | Protein: 5g | Fat: 20g | Net Carbs: 7g | Fiber: 2g

Key Benefits: Cauliflower provides fiber and vitamins, while leeks add flavor and antioxidants.

Recipe Modification: Top with grated Parmesan cheese or crispy bacon bits.

GREEK SALAD WITH GRILLED CHICKEN

Servings: 2-3

Prep Time: 15 minutes

Cook Time: 15 minutes

Ingredients:

- 2 boneless, skinless chicken breasts
- 6 cups mixed salad greens
- 1 cup cucumber, diced
- 1 cup cherry tomatoes, halved
- 1/4 cup sliced red onion
- 1/4 cup crumbled feta cheese
- 2 tablespoons chopped fresh oregano
- 2 tablespoons olive oil
- Juice of 1 lemon
- Salt and pepper to taste

Instructions:

1. Preheat a grill or grill pan.
2. Season chicken breasts with chopped fresh oregano, olive oil, salt, and pepper.
3. Grill chicken for about 6-7 minutes per side or until cooked through.
4. Slice grilled chicken into strips.
5. In a large salad bowl, combine mixed salad greens, diced cucumber, halved cherry tomatoes, sliced red onion, and crumbled feta cheese.
6. Add sliced grilled chicken on top.
7. Drizzle with olive oil and lemon juice.
8. Toss gently to combine.
9. Serve as a Mediterranean-inspired salad.

Nutritional Information:

Calories: 300 (per serving) | Protein: 25g | Fat: 15g | Net Carbs: 8g | Fiber: 3g

Key Benefits: Grilled chicken provides protein, while mixed greens offer vitamins and minerals.

Recipe Modification: Add Kalamata olives for extra Greek flair.

CREAMY MUSHROOM SOUP

Servings: 4-6

Prep Time: 10 minutes

Cook Time: 25 minutes

Ingredients:

- 2 cups sliced mushrooms
- 1 small onion, diced
- 2 cloves garlic, minced
- 4 cups chicken or vegetable broth
- 1 cup heavy cream
- 2 tablespoons butter
- 2 tablespoons chopped fresh thyme
- Salt and pepper to taste

Instructions:

1. In a pot, melt butter and sauté diced onion and minced garlic until translucent.
2. Add sliced mushrooms and cook until browned.
3. Pour in chicken or vegetable broth and bring to a simmer.
4. Let the soup simmer for about 15-20 minutes.
5. Use an immersion blender to puree the soup until smooth.
6. Stir in heavy cream and chopped fresh thyme.

7. Season with salt and pepper. Serve hot.

Nutritional Information:

Calories: 300 (per serving) | Protein: 5g | Fat: 25g | Net Carbs: 7g | Fiber: 1g

Key Benefits: Mushrooms provide vitamins and minerals, while thyme adds flavor and antioxidants.

Recipe Modification: Garnish with a drizzle of truffle oil for a luxurious touch.

COBB SALAD WITH RANCH DRESSING

Servings: 2-3

Prep Time: 15 minutes

Ingredients:

- 2 cups cooked and diced chicken breast
- 6 cups mixed salad greens
- 1 cup diced cucumber
- 1/2 cup crumbled blue cheese
- 1/4 cup diced tomatoes
- 1/4 cup diced cooked bacon
- 2 hard-boiled eggs, sliced
- 1/4 cup diced red onion
- 2 tablespoons chopped fresh chives
- Salt and pepper to taste
- Ranch dressing for drizzling

Instructions:

1. In a large salad bowl, combine diced cooked chicken breast, mixed salad greens, diced cucumber, crumbled blue cheese, diced tomatoes, diced cooked bacon, sliced hard-boiled eggs, diced red onion, and chopped fresh chives.
2. Drizzle with ranch dressing.
3. Toss gently to combine.

4. Serve as a hearty and flavorful salad.

Nutritional Information:

Calories: 350 (per serving) | Protein: 25g | Fat: 20g | Net Carbs: 9g | Fiber: 3g

Key Benefits: Chicken provides protein, while blue cheese adds richness and flavor.

Recipe Modification: Substitute turkey bacon for a leaner option.

ROASTED RED PEPPER AND TOMATO SOUP

Servings: 4-6

Prep Time: 15 minutes

Cook Time: 30 minutes

Ingredients:

- 2 red bell peppers, roasted and peeled
- 4 cups diced tomatoes (canned or fresh)
- 1 small onion, diced
- 2 cloves garlic, minced
- 4 cups chicken or vegetable broth
- 1/2 cup heavy cream
- 2 tablespoons olive oil
- Salt and pepper to taste
- Fresh basil leaves for garnish

Instructions:

1. Preheat the oven to 400°F (200°C).
2. Place red bell peppers on a baking sheet and roast in the oven until the skin is charred.
3. Remove the peppers from the oven and place them in a bowl covered with plastic wrap. This will make it easier to peel the skin.
4. Once cooled, peel the skin off the peppers and dice them.
5. In a pot, heat olive oil and sauté diced onion and minced garlic until translucent.
6. Add diced tomatoes and diced roasted red peppers, and cook for a few minutes.

7. Pour in chicken or vegetable broth and bring to a simmer.
8. Let the soup simmer for about 15-20 minutes.
9. Use an immersion blender to puree the soup until smooth.
10. Stir in heavy cream and season with salt and pepper.
11. Serve hot, garnished with fresh basil leaves.

Nutritional Information:

Calories: 250 (per serving) | Protein: 5g | Fat: 20g | Net Carbs: 9g | Fiber: 2g

Key Benefits: Red bell peppers provide vitamins and antioxidants, while tomatoes add rich flavor.

Recipe Modification: Top with a drizzle of balsamic reduction for extra sweetness.

AVOCADO CUCUMBER SALAD

Servings: 2-3

Prep Time: 10 minutes

Ingredients:

- 2 ripe avocados, diced
- 1 cucumber, diced
- 1/4 cup diced red onion
- 2 tablespoons chopped fresh cilantro
- Juice of 1 lime
- 2 tablespoons olive oil
- Salt and pepper to taste

Instructions:

1. In a bowl, combine diced avocado, diced cucumber, and diced red onion, chopped cilantro, lime juice, olive oil, salt, and pepper.
2. Toss gently to combine.
3. Serve as a refreshing and nutritious salad.

Nutritional Information:

Calories: 200 (per serving) | Protein: 2g | Fat: 18g | Net Carbs: 7g | Fiber: 5g

Key Benefits: Avocado offers healthy fats and vitamins, while cucumber provides hydration.

Recipe Modification: Add diced tomatoes or bell peppers for extra color and flavor.

SPINACH AND STRAWBERRY SALAD

Servings: 2-3

Prep Time: 10 minutes

Ingredients:

- 6 cups baby spinach leaves
- 1 cup sliced strawberries
- 1/4 cup crumbled goat cheese
- 1/4 cup chopped walnuts
- 2 tablespoons balsamic vinegar
- 2 tablespoons olive oil
- 1 teaspoon honey (optional)
- Salt and pepper to taste

Instructions:

1. In a large salad bowl, combine baby spinach leaves, sliced strawberries, crumbled goat cheese, and chopped walnuts.
2. In a small bowl, whisk together balsamic vinegar, olive oil, honey (if using), salt, and pepper to make the dressing.
3. Drizzle the dressing over the salad.
4. Toss gently to combine.
5. Serve as a sweet and savory salad.

Nutritional Information:

Calories: 250 (per serving) | Protein: 5g | Fat: 20g | Net Carbs: 9g | Fiber: 3g

Key Benefits: Spinach offers vitamins and antioxidants, while strawberries add natural sweetness.

Recipe Modification: Substitute honey with a low-carb sweetener for a keto-friendly version

---

LEMON CHICKEN ORZO SOUP

Servings: 4-6

Prep Time: 15 minutes

Cook Time: 25 minutes

Ingredients:

- 2 cups diced cooked chicken breast
- 1 cup orzo pasta
- 4 cups chicken broth
- 2 cups chopped spinach leaves
- Juice of 2 lemons
- 2 cloves garlic, minced
- 1 small onion, diced
- 2 tablespoons olive oil
- Salt and pepper to taste
- Chopped fresh parsley for garnish

Instructions:

1. In a pot, heat olive oil and sauté diced onion and minced garlic until translucent.
2. Add orzo pasta and cook for a few minutes.
3. Pour in chicken broth and bring to a boil.
4. Let the soup simmer for about 10-12 minutes or until the orzo is cooked.
5. Stir in diced cooked chicken breast, chopped spinach leaves, and lemon juice.
6. Season with salt and pepper.
7. Serve hot, garnished with chopped fresh parsley.

Nutritional Information:

Calories: 300 (per serving) | Protein: 20g | Fat: 10g | Net Carbs: 8g | Fiber: 2g

Key Benefits: Chicken provides protein, while spinach offers vitamins and minerals.

Recipe Modification: Add a sprinkle of grated Parmesan cheese before serving.

ZUCCHINI NOODLE SALAD WITH PESTO DRESSING

Servings: 2-3

Prep Time: 15 minutes

Ingredients:

- 2 large zucchinis, spiralized into noodles
- 1 cup cherry tomatoes, halved
- 1/4 cup crumbled feta cheese
- 1/4 cup chopped fresh basil
- 1/4 cup chopped walnuts
- 2 tablespoons olive oil
- 2 tablespoons pesto sauce
- Juice of 1 lemon
- Salt and pepper to taste

Instructions:

1. In a bowl, combine zucchini noodle strands, halved cherry tomatoes, crumbled feta cheese, chopped fresh basil, and chopped walnuts.
2. In a small bowl, whisk together olive oil, pesto sauce, lemon juice, salt, and pepper to make the dressing.
3. Drizzle the dressing over the salad.
4. Toss gently to combine.
5. Serve as a light and flavorful salad.

Nutritional Information:

Calories: 250 (per serving) | Protein: 5g | Fat: 20g | Net Carbs: 7g | Fiber: 3g

Key Benefits: Zucchini noodles provide a low-carb base, while pesto adds vibrant flavor.

Recipe Modification: Add grilled chicken or shrimp for extra protein.

POULTRY AND SEAFOOD RECIPES

PESTO GRILLED SALMON

Servings: 2

Prep Time: 10 minutes

Cook Time: 10 minutes

Ingredients:

- 2 salmon fillets
- Salt and pepper, to taste
- 1/4 cup pesto sauce (sugar-free)
- Lemon wedges, for serving

Instructions:

1. Preheat the grill.
2. Season salmon fillets with salt and pepper.
3. Grill salmon until cooked to desired doneness.
4. Brush salmon with pesto sauce during the last few minutes of grilling.
5. Serve with lemon wedges.
6. Enjoy your delicious pesto grilled salmon!

Nutritional Information:

Calories: 350 | Protein: 30g | Fat: 22g | Net Carbs: 2g | Fiber: 1g

Benefits: Salmon provides omega-3 fatty acids, and pesto adds vibrant flavor.

Recipe Modification: Add roasted cherry tomatoes on top for extra color.

CREAMY GARLIC PARMESAN CHICKEN

Servings: 2

Prep Time: 10 minutes

Cook Time: 20 minutes

Ingredients:

- 2 boneless, skinless chicken breasts
- Salt and pepper, to taste
- 2 tbsps. olive oil
- 2 cloves garlic, minced
- 1/2 cup heavy cream
- 1/4 cup grated Parmesan cheese
- Chopped fresh parsley, for garnish

Instructions:

1. Season chicken breasts with salt and pepper.
2. In a pan, heat olive oil and cook chicken until browned and cooked through.
3. Remove chicken from the pan and set aside.
4. In the same pan, sauté minced garlic until fragrant.
5. Add heavy cream and grated Parmesan cheese, and stir until smooth.
6. Return chicken to the pan and simmer in the sauce for a few minutes.
7. Garnish with chopped parsley.
8. Enjoy your creamy garlic Parmesan chicken!

Nutritional Information:

Calories: 400Protein: 30g | Fat: 28g | Net Carbs: 3g | Fiber: 0g

Benefits: Chicken provides protein, and Parmesan adds richness.

Recipe Modification: Add chopped sun-dried tomatoes for extra flavor.

COCONUT LIME GRILLED CHICKEN

Servings: 2

Prep Time: 10 minutes

Cook Time: 15 minutes

Ingredients:

- 2 boneless, skinless chicken breasts
- Salt and pepper, to taste
- Zest and juice of 1 lime
- 1/4 cup coconut milk
- 1 teaspoon curry powder (optional)
- Fresh cilantro, for garnish

Instructions:

1. Preheat the grill.
2. Season chicken breasts with salt, pepper, and curry powder (if using).
3. In a bowl, mix lime zest, lime juice, and coconut milk.
4. Marinate chicken in the lime-coconut mixture for about 10 minutes.
5. Grill chicken until cooked through.
6. Garnish with fresh cilantro.
7. Enjoy your tropical coconut lime grilled chicken!

Nutritional Information:

Calories: 300 | Protein: 30g | Fat: 16g | Net Carbs: 2g | Fiber: 0g

Benefits: Chicken offers lean protein, and coconut milk adds creaminess.

Recipe Modification: Add a touch of grated ginger to the marinade for extra zest.

HERB-CRUSTED BAKED COD

Servings: 2

Prep Time: 10 minutes

Cook Time: 15 minutes

Ingredients:

- 2 cod fillets
- Salt and pepper, to taste
- 2 tbsps. olive oil
- 1/4 cup almond flour
- 1 teaspoon dried herbs (e.g., thyme, rosemary)
- Lemon wedges, for serving

Instructions:

1. Preheat the oven to 400°F (200°C).
2. Season cod fillets with salt and pepper.
3. In a bowl, mix almond flour and dried herbs.
4. Brush cod fillets with olive oil, then coat with the almond flour mixture.
5. Place cod fillets on a baking sheet.
6. Bake for about 12-15 minutes, until fish flakes easily.
7. Serve with lemon wedges.
8. Enjoy your herb-crusted baked cod!

Nutritional Information:

Calories: 250 | Protein: 25g | Fat: 15g | Net Carbs: 3g | Fiber: 2g

Benefits: Cod offers lean protein, and almond flour adds a crispy crust.

Recipe Modification: Add a pinch of garlic powder for extra flavor.

CAJUN GRILLED TURKEY BREAST

Servings: 2

Prep Time: 10 minutes

Cook Time: 20 minutes

Ingredients:

- 2 turkey breast cutlets
- Salt and pepper, to taste
- 1 tbsps. olive oil
- 1 teaspoon Cajun seasoning
- Lime wedges, for serving

Instructions:

1. Preheat the grill.
2. Season turkey cutlets with salt, pepper, and Cajun seasoning.
3. Brush cutlets with olive oil.
4. Grill turkey until cooked through.
5. Serve with lime wedges.
6. Enjoy your flavorful Cajun grilled turkey!

Nutritional Information:

Calories: 220 | Protein: 30g | Fat: 10g | Net Carbs: 1g | Fiber: 0g

Benefits: Turkey offers lean protein, and Cajun seasoning adds a kick.

Recipe Modification: Use chicken breast if preferred.

CREAMY TUSCAN SHRIMP

Servings: 2

Prep Time: 10 minutes

Cook Time: 15 minutes

Ingredients:

- 8 oz. shrimp, peeled and deveined
- Salt and pepper, to taste
- 2 tbsps. butter
- 2 cloves garlic, minced
- 1/2 cup heavy cream
- 1/4 cup sun-dried tomatoes, chopped
- 1 cup fresh spinach
- Grated Parmesan cheese, for garnish

Instructions:

1. Season shrimp with salt and pepper.
2. In a pan, melt butter and sauté minced garlic until fragrant.
3. Add shrimp and cook until pink and opaque.
4. Remove shrimp from the pan and set aside.
5. In the same pan, add heavy cream and chopped sun-dried tomatoes.
6. Simmer until the sauce thickens.
7. Add fresh spinach and stir until wilted.
8. Return shrimp to the pan and warm through.
9. Serve with a sprinkle of grated Parmesan cheese.
10. Enjoy your creamy Tuscan shrimp!

Nutritional Information:

Calories: 350 | Protein: 25g | Fat: 26g | Net Carbs: 6g | Fiber: 1g

Benefits: Shrimp offers protein, and spinach adds vitamins and color.

Recipe Modification: Add a splash of white wine to the sauce for extra flavor.

ROSEMARY ROASTED CHICKEN THIGHS

Servings: 2

Prep Time: 10 minutes

Cook Time: 35 minutes

Ingredients:

- 4 bone-in, skin-on chicken thighs
- Salt and pepper, to taste
- 2 tbsps. olive oil
- 2 sprigs fresh rosemary
- Lemon wedges, for serving

Instructions:

1. Preheat the oven to 400°F (200°C).
2. Season chicken thighs with salt and pepper.
3. In a pan, heat olive oil.
4. Sear chicken thighs, skin side down, until golden brown.
5. Flip chicken thighs and add fresh rosemary sprigs.
6. Transfer the pan to the oven and roast for about 25-30 minutes, until cooked through.
7. Serve with lemon wedges.
8. Enjoy your rosemary roasted chicken thighs!

Nutritional Information:

Calories: 400 | Protein: 25g | Fat: 32g | Net Carbs: 0g | Fiber: 0g

Benefits: Chicken thighs provide protein and healthy fats, while rosemary adds aromatic flavor.

Recipe Modification: Add minced garlic to the olive oil for extra depth.

SEARED TUNA STEAK WITH AVOCADO SALSA

Servings: 2

Prep Time: 15 minutes

Cook Time: 5 minutes

Ingredients:

- 2 tuna steak fillets
- Salt and pepper, to taste
- 2 tbsps. olive oil
- 1 ripe avocado, diced
- 1/4 cup diced red onion
- 1/4 cup diced tomato
- Fresh cilantro, chopped
- Lime juice, to taste

Instructions:

1. Season tuna steak fillets with salt and pepper.
2. In a pan, heat olive oil over high heat.
3. Sear tuna steaks for about 1-2 minutes on each side for medium-rare.
4. In a bowl, combine diced avocado, red onion, tomato, chopped cilantro, and lime juice.
5. Serve seared tuna with avocado salsa on top.
6. Enjoy your refreshing seared tuna steak with avocado salsa!

Nutritional Information:

Calories: 300 | Protein: 30g | Fat: 18g | Net Carbs: 6g | Fiber: 4g

Benefits: Tuna offers protein and omega-3 fatty acids, while avocado provides healthy fats and vitamins.

Recipe Modification: Add a touch of chopped jalapeño for extra heat

SIDE DISHES

SPICED CABBAGE AND CARROT SLAW

Servings: 2-3

Prep Time: 15 minutes

Cook Time: 0 minutes

Ingredients:

- 3 cups shredded cabbage
- 1 cup shredded carrots
- 1/4 cup chopped fresh parsley
- 2 tablespoons olive oil
- 1 tablespoon apple cider vinegar
- 1 teaspoon ground cumin
- 1/2 teaspoon ground coriander
- 1/4 teaspoon ground turmeric
- Salt and pepper to taste

Instructions:

1. In a large bowl, combine shredded cabbage, shredded carrots, and chopped fresh parsley.
2. In a small bowl, whisk together olive oil, apple cider vinegar, ground cumin, ground coriander, ground turmeric, salt, and pepper.
3. Drizzle the dressing over the cabbage and carrot mixture. Toss to coat.
4. Serve spiced cabbage and carrot slaw as a vibrant and flavorful side.

Nutritional Information:

Calories: 100 (per serving) | Protein: 2g | Fat: 8g | Net Carbs: 6g | Fiber: 3g

Key Benefits: Cabbage and carrots offer vitamins and antioxidants, while spices add depth.

Recipe Modification: Add a sprinkle of toasted pumpkin seeds for extra crunch.

BROCCOLI AND ALMOND STIR-FRY

Servings: 2-3

Prep Time: 10 minutes

Cook Time: 10 minutes

Ingredients:

- 2 cups broccoli florets
- 1/4 cup sliced almonds
- 2 tablespoons olive oil
- 1 tablespoon soy sauce (or tamari for gluten-free)
- 1 teaspoon sesame oil
- 1 teaspoon minced fresh ginger
- Salt and pepper to taste

Instructions:

1. In a skillet, heat olive oil and sauté broccoli florets until slightly tender.
2. Add sliced almonds and sauté until they are lightly toasted.
3. Stir in soy sauce, sesame oil, minced fresh ginger, salt, and pepper.
4. Cook for another minute to combine flavors.
5. Serve broccoli and almond stir-fry as a crunchy and satisfying side.

Nutritional Information:

Calories: 150 (per serving) | Protein: 4g | Fat: 12g | Net Carbs: 6g | Fiber: 3g

Key Benefits: Broccoli provides fiber and vitamins, while almonds offer healthy fats.

Recipe Modification: Add a sprinkle of red pepper flakes for some heat.

GARLIC ROASTED ASPARAGUS

Servings: 2-3

Prep Time: 5 minutes

Cook Time: 15 minutes

Ingredients:

- 1 bunch asparagus, trimmed
- 2 tablespoons olive oil
- 3 cloves garlic, minced
- Salt and pepper to taste

Instructions:

1. Preheat the oven to 400°F (200°C).
2. Toss asparagus with olive oil, minced garlic, salt, and pepper.
3. Spread asparagus on a baking sheet in a single layer.
4. Roast in the oven for about 12-15 minutes or until tender and slightly crispy.
5. Serve hot as a flavorful and nutritious side dish.

Nutritional Information:

Calories: 100 (per serving) | Protein: 2g | Fat: 8g | Net Carbs: 4g | Fiber: 2g

Key Benefits: Asparagus is rich in vitamins and antioxidants, while garlic adds flavor.

Recipe Modification: Sprinkle grated Parmesan cheese over the roasted asparagus for extra indulgence.

CAULIFLOWER MASH WITH GARLIC AND CHIVES

Servings: 2-3

Prep Time: 10 minutes

Cook Time: 15 minutes

Ingredients:

- 1 medium head cauliflower, cut into florets
- 2 cloves garlic, minced
- 2 tablespoons butter
- 2 tablespoons chopped fresh chives
- Salt and pepper to taste

Instructions:

1. Steam or boil cauliflower florets until tender.
2. Drain cauliflower and transfer to a food processor.
3. Add minced garlic, butter, chopped fresh chives, salt, and pepper.
4. Blend until smooth and creamy.
5. Serve cauliflower mash as a low-carb alternative to mashed potatoes.

Nutritional Information:

Calories: 150 (per serving) | Protein: 4g | Fat: 10g | Net Carbs: 6g | Fiber: 3g

Key Benefits: Cauliflower provides vitamins and fiber, while chives add freshness.

Recipe Modification: Blend in some cream cheese for extra creaminess.

CABBAGE AND RADISH SLAW

Servings: 2-3

Prep Time: 15 minutes

Cook Time: 0 minutes

Ingredients:

- 3 cups shredded cabbage
- 1 cup sliced radishes
- 1/4 cup chopped fresh cilantro
- 2 tablespoons mayonnaise
- 1 tablespoon apple cider vinegar
- 1 teaspoon Dijon mustard
- Salt and pepper to taste

Instructions:

1. In a large bowl, combine shredded cabbage, sliced radishes, and chopped fresh cilantro.
2. In a small bowl, whisk together mayonnaise, apple cider vinegar, Dijon mustard, salt, and pepper.
3. Drizzle the dressing over the cabbage and radish mixture. Toss to coat.
4. Serve cabbage and radish slaw as a crisp and tangy side.

Nutritional Information:

Calories: 150 (per serving) | Protein: 2g | Fat: 12g | Net Carbs: 6g | Fiber: 3g

Key Benefits: Cabbage provides fiber and antioxidants, while radishes add crunch.

Recipe Modification: Add toasted sunflower seeds for extra texture.

MUSHROOM AND SPINACH SAUTÉ

Servings: 2-3

Prep Time: 10 minutes

Cook Time: 10 minutes

Ingredients:

- 2 cups sliced mushrooms
- 2 cups fresh spinach leaves
- 2 cloves garlic, minced
- 2 tablespoons butter
- Salt and pepper to taste

Instructions:

1. In a skillet, melt butter over medium heat.
2. Sauté sliced mushrooms until they release their moisture and are cooked down.
3. Add minced garlic and sauté until fragrant.
4. Stir in fresh spinach leaves and cook until wilted.
5. Season with salt and pepper.
6. Serve mushroom and spinach sauté as a flavorful and nutrient-rich side.

Nutritional Information:

Calories: 100 (per serving) | Protein: 4g | Fat: 8g | Net Carbs: 4g | Fiber: 2g

Key Benefits: Mushrooms offer vitamins and minerals, while spinach adds nutrients.

Recipe Modification: Drizzle with lemon juice for extra zest.

ROASTED EGGPLANT WITH TAHINI DRIZZLE

Servings: 2-3

Prep Time: 10 minutes

Cook Time: 25 minutes

Ingredients:

- 1 medium eggplant, sliced
- 2 tablespoons olive oil
- 2 tablespoons tahini
- 1 tablespoon lemon juice
- 1 clove garlic, minced
- Chopped fresh parsley (for garnish)
- Salt and pepper to taste

Instructions:

1. Preheat the oven to 400°F (200°C).
2. Place eggplant slices on a baking sheet and drizzle with olive oil. Season with salt and pepper.
3. Roast eggplant slices in the oven for about 20-25 minutes or until they are tender and golden.
4. In a bowl, whisk together tahini, lemon juice, minced garlic, salt, and pepper.
5. Drizzle the tahini mixture over the roasted eggplant slices.
6. Garnish with chopped fresh parsley before serving.

Nutritional Information:

Calories: 150 (per serving) | Protein: 2g | Fat: 12g | Net Carbs: 6g | Fiber: 3g

Key Benefits: Eggplant offers antioxidants, while tahini provides healthy fats.

Recipe Modification: Sprinkle with toasted sesame seeds for added crunch.

GREEN BEAN AND CHERRY TOMATO SALAD

Servings: 2-3

Prep Time: 10 minutes

Cook Time: 5 minutes

Ingredients:

- 2 cups trimmed green beans
- 1 cup cherry tomatoes, halved
- 1/4 cup crumbled feta cheese
- 2 tablespoons chopped fresh basil
- 2 tablespoons olive oil
- 1 tablespoon balsamic vinegar
- Salt and pepper to taste

Instructions:

1. Steam or blanch green beans until they are crisp-tender. Rinse under cold water and drain.
2. In a bowl, combine trimmed green beans, halved cherry tomatoes, crumbled feta cheese, and chopped fresh basil.
3. Drizzle olive oil and balsamic vinegar over the mixture.
4. Add salt and pepper. Gently toss to combine.
5. Serve green bean and cherry tomato salad as a vibrant and balanced side.

Nutritional Information:

Calories: 150 (per serving) | Protein: 4g | Fat: 10g | Net Carbs: 8g | Fiber: 3g

Key Benefits: Green beans provide vitamins and fiber, while tomatoes add antioxidants.

Recipe Modification: Substitute goat cheese for feta cheese if desired.

VEGETARIAN ENTREES

CAULIFLOWER AND BROCCOLI RICE STIR-FRY

Servings: 2

Prep Time: 15 minutes

Cook Time: 10 minutes

Ingredients:

- 2 cups cauliflower rice
- 1 cup broccoli florets
- 1 cup sliced bell peppers
- 1/2 cup sliced carrots
- 2 cloves garlic, minced
- 2 tablespoons low-sodium soy sauce (or tamari for gluten-free)
- 1 tablespoon olive oil
- 1 teaspoon sesame oil
- 1 teaspoon grated fresh ginger
- 1/4 cup chopped scallions
- Salt and pepper to taste

Instructions:

1. In a large skillet, heat olive oil and sauté minced garlic and grated fresh ginger until fragrant.
2. Add sliced bell peppers and sliced carrots. Sauté until slightly softened.
3. Stir in cauliflower rice and broccoli florets. Cook for a few minutes until tender.
4. Drizzle low-sodium soy sauce and sesame oil over the mixture. Toss to combine.
5. Season with salt and pepper.
6. Serve hot, garnished with chopped scallions.

Nutritional Information:

Calories: 200 (per serving) | Protein: 6g | Fat: 10g | Net Carbs: 10g | Fiber: 5g

Key Benefits: Cauliflower and broccoli provide fiber and vitamins, while sesame and ginger add flavor.

Recipe Modification: Add tofu or tempeh for extra protein.

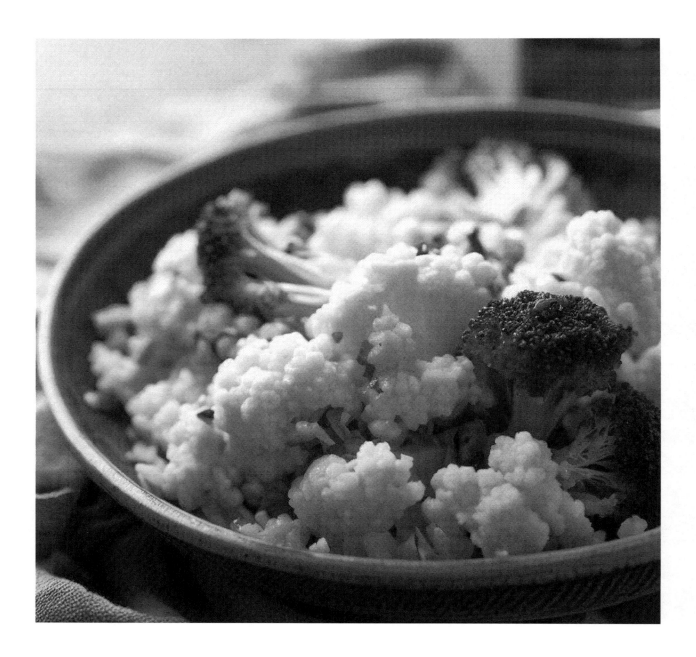

EGGPLANT AND MUSHROOM RATATOUILLE

Servings: 2-3

Prep Time: 20 minutes

Cook Time: 25 minutes

Ingredients:

- 1 medium eggplant, diced
- 1 cup sliced mushrooms
- 1 cup diced zucchini
- 1 cup diced bell peppers
- 1 cup diced tomatoes (canned or fresh)
- 2 cloves garlic, minced
- 2 tablespoons olive oil
- 1 teaspoon dried thyme
- 1 teaspoon dried oregano
- Salt and pepper to taste

Instructions:

1. In a skillet, heat olive oil and sauté diced eggplant until slightly softened.
2. Add sliced mushrooms and diced zucchini. Sauté until vegetables are tender.
3. Stir in diced bell peppers, diced tomatoes, minced garlic, dried thyme, dried oregano, salt, and pepper.
4. Cook for another 5-7 minutes to meld the flavors.
5. Serve hot as a stew or over cauliflower rice.

Nutritional Information:

Calories: 150 (per serving) | Protein: 4g | Fat: 10g | Net Carbs: 12g | Fiber: 5g

Key Benefits: Eggplant and mushrooms provide antioxidants, while various vegetables add a range of nutrients.

Tips: Top with fresh basil or parsley for a burst of freshness.

PORTOBELLO MUSHROOM AND GOAT CHEESE STUFFED SQUASH

Servings: 2-3

Prep Time: 20 minutes

Cook Time: 30 minutes

Ingredients:

- 3 small acorn squashes, halved and seeds removed
- 3 large Portobello mushrooms, diced
- 1/2 cup crumbled goat cheese
- 1/4 cup chopped walnuts
- 1/4 cup chopped fresh parsley
- 2 tablespoons olive oil
- 1 teaspoon dried thyme
- Salt and pepper to taste

Instructions:

1. Preheat the oven to 375°F (190°C).
2. Place acorn squash halves on a baking dish and drizzle with olive oil. Season with salt and pepper.
3. Roast squash halves in the oven for about 20-25 minutes or until they are tender.
4. In a skillet, heat olive oil and sauté diced Portobello mushrooms until softened.
5. Stir in crumbled goat cheese, chopped walnuts, chopped fresh parsley, dried thyme, salt, and pepper.
6. Once the squash halves are roasted, stuff them with the Portobello mushroom and goat cheese mixture.
7. Return stuffed squash halves to the oven and bake for an additional 10-15 minutes.
8. Serve hot as a delightful and hearty vegetarian entrée.

Nutritional Information:

Calories: 300 (per serving) | Protein: 8g | Fat: 20g | Net Carbs: 20g | Fiber: 6g

Key Benefits: Acorn squash is rich in vitamins, while Portobello mushrooms and goat cheese provide flavor and protein.

Recipe Modification: Use different types of cheese or nuts for variation.

CHICKPEA AND SPINACH COCONUT CURRY

Servings: 2-3

Prep Time: 15 minutes

Cook Time: 25 minutes

Ingredients:

- 2 cups cooked chickpeas (canned or soaked and boiled)
- 2 cups fresh spinach leaves
- 1 can (14 ounces) coconut milk
- 1 onion, finely chopped
- 2 cloves garlic, minced
- 1 tablespoon curry powder
- 1 teaspoon ground turmeric
- 1 teaspoon ground cumin
- 1 teaspoon paprika
- 1 tablespoon olive oil
- Salt and pepper to taste
- Chopped fresh cilantro (for garnish)

Instructions:

1. In a skillet, heat olive oil and sauté finely chopped onion and minced garlic until translucent.
2. Stir in curry powder, ground turmeric, ground cumin, and paprika. Cook for a minute.
3. Add cooked chickpeas and fresh spinach leaves. Sauté until spinach wilts.
4. Pour in coconut milk and let the mixture simmer for about 10-15 minutes.
5. Season with salt and pepper.

6. Serve hot, garnished with chopped fresh cilantro.

Nutritional Information:

Calories: 300 (per serving) | Protein: 10g | Fat: 15g | Net Carbs: 20g | Fiber: 6g

Key Benefits: Chickpeas offer protein and fiber, while spinach adds nutrients.

Tips: Serve over cauliflower rice for a low-carb option.

SPAGHETTI SQUASH WITH PESTO AND ROASTED TOMATOES

Servings: 2-3

Prep Time: 15 minutes

Cook Time: 40 minutes

Ingredients:

- 1 medium spaghetti squash
- 1 cup cherry tomatoes
- 1/4 cup pesto sauce
- 2 tablespoons olive oil
- 1/4 cup grated Parmesan cheese
- Salt and pepper to taste
- Chopped fresh basil (for garnish)

Instructions:

1. Preheat the oven to 375°F (190°C).
2. Cut spaghetti squash in half lengthwise and remove seeds.
3. Brush the cut sides with olive oil and season with salt and pepper.
4. Place spaghetti squash halves cut-side down on a baking sheet.
5. Roast in the oven for about 30-35 minutes or until the strands can be easily separated with a fork.
6. In the meantime, toss cherry tomatoes with olive oil, salt, and pepper. Place them on a separate baking sheet.
7. Roast the tomatoes in the oven for about 10-15 minutes or until they burst and caramelize.

8. Use a fork to separate the spaghetti squash strands.
9. Toss the strands with pesto sauce.
10. Serve hot, topped with roasted tomatoes, grated Parmesan cheese, and chopped fresh basil.

Nutritional Information:

Calories: 250 (per serving) | Protein: 6g | Fat: 20g | Net Carbs: 15g | Fiber: 4g

Key Benefits: Spaghetti squash is low in calories and carbs, while pesto and tomatoes add flavor.

Recipe Modification: Add roasted pine nuts for extra crunch.

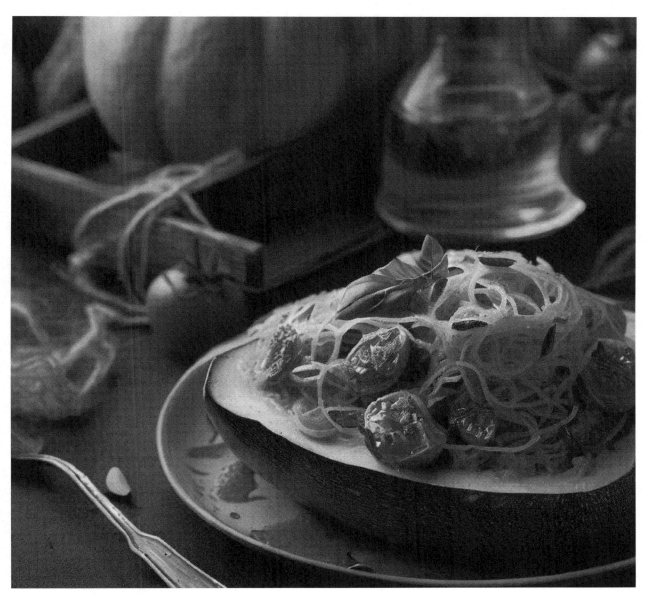

BRUSSELS SPROUTS AND PECAN SALAD

Servings: 2-3

Prep Time: 15 minutes

Cook Time: 15 minutes

Ingredients:

- 4 cups shaved Brussels sprouts
- 1/2 cup chopped pecans
- 1/4 cup crumbled blue cheese
- 1/4 cup dried cranberries
- 2 tablespoons olive oil
- 2 tablespoons balsamic vinegar
- 1 tablespoon Dijon mustard
- Salt and pepper to taste

Instructions:

1. In a skillet, toast chopped pecans over medium heat until fragrant and lightly browned. Set aside.
2. In a bowl, whisk together olive oil, balsamic vinegar, Dijon mustard, salt, and pepper to make the dressing.
3. Toss shaved Brussels sprouts with the dressing.
4. Fold in toasted pecans, crumbled blue cheese, and dried cranberries.
5. Serve the salad as a nutrient-packed and flavorful entrée.

Nutritional Information:

Calories: 250 (per serving) | Protein: 6g | Fat: 20g | Net Carbs: 15g | Fiber: 6g

Key Benefits: Brussels sprouts provide vitamins and fiber, while pecans offer healthy fats.

Recipe Modification: Add grilled tofu or tempeh for extra protein.

CAULIFLOWER AND SPINACH CURRY

Servings: 2-3

Prep Time: 15 minutes

Cook Time: 25 minutes

Ingredients:

- 1 medium cauliflower, cut into florets
- 2 cups fresh spinach leaves
- 1 can (14 ounces) coconut milk
- 1 onion, finely chopped
- 2 cloves garlic, minced
- 1 tablespoon curry powder
- 1 teaspoon ground turmeric
- 1 teaspoon ground cumin
- 1 teaspoon ground coriander
- 2 tablespoons olive oil
- Salt and pepper to taste
- Chopped fresh cilantro (for garnish)

Instructions:

1. In a skillet, heat olive oil and sauté finely chopped onion and minced garlic until translucent.
2. Stir in curry powder, ground turmeric, ground cumin, and ground coriander. Cook for a minute.
3. Add cauliflower florets and sauté until slightly softened.
4. Stir in fresh spinach leaves and let them wilt.
5. Pour in coconut milk and let the mixture simmer for about 10-15 minutes.
6. Season with salt and pepper.
7. Serve hot, garnished with chopped fresh cilantro.

Nutritional Information:

Calories: 250 (per serving) | Protein: 6g | Fat: 20g | Net Carbs: 15g | Fiber: 6g

Key Benefits: Cauliflower provides vitamins and fiber, while coconut milk adds creaminess.

Recipe Modification: Serve over cauliflower rice or with a side of roasted nuts.

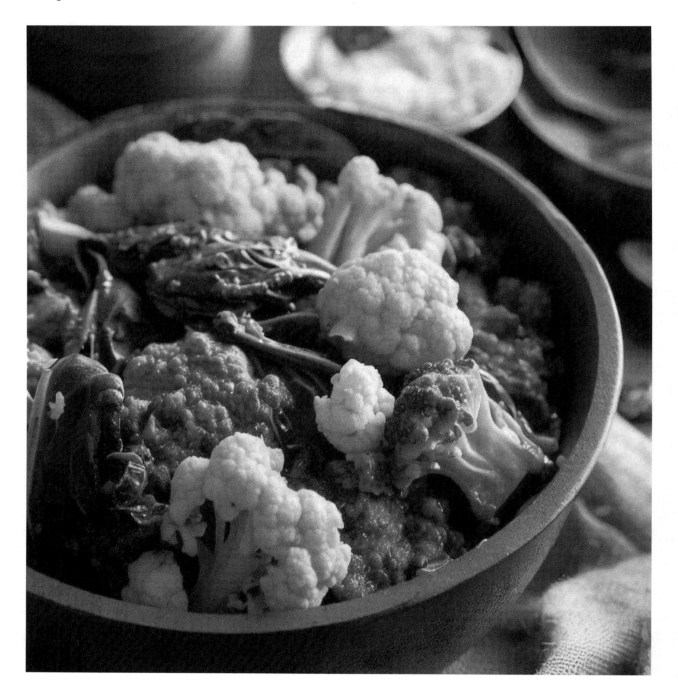

DESSERT

STRAWBERRY CHIA SEED PUDDING

Servings: 2-3

Prep Time: 10 minutes

Cook Time: 0 minutes (plus chilling time)

Ingredients:

- 1 cup unsweetened almond milk
- 1 cup fresh strawberries, hulled
- 1/4 cup chia seeds
- 2 tablespoons low-carb sweetener (such as stevia)
- 1 teaspoon vanilla extract

Instructions:

1. In a blender, combine almond milk, fresh strawberries, low-carb sweetener, and vanilla extract. Blend until smooth.
2. Pour the strawberry mixture into a bowl and stir in chia seeds.
3. Cover and refrigerate for at least 3 hours or until the chia seeds have absorbed the liquid and the mixture has thickened.
4. Stir the pudding before serving and divide into individual cups.

Nutritional Information:

Calories: 150 (per serving) | Protein: 4g | Fat: 8g | Net Carbs: 8g | Fiber: 12g

Key Benefits: Chia seeds provide fiber and omega-3 fatty acids, while strawberries add vitamins and antioxidants.

Recipe Modification: Add a dollop of whipped coconut cream on top.

COCONUT LIME PANNA COTTA

Servings: 2-3

Prep Time: 15 minutes

Cook Time: 10 minutes (plus chilling time)

Ingredients:

- 1 cup unsweetened coconut milk
- 1/2 cup heavy cream
- 1/4 cup low-carb sweetener (such as erythritol)
- Zest and juice of 1 lime
- 1 teaspoon gelatin powder
- 1 tablespoon cold water
- Fresh mint leaves (for garnish)

Instructions:

1. In a saucepan, combine unsweetened coconut milk, heavy cream, low-carb sweetener, lime zest, and lime juice. Heat over medium heat until it starts to simmer. Remove from heat.
2. In a small bowl, sprinkle gelatin powder over cold water and let it bloom for a few minutes.
3. Add the bloomed gelatin mixture to the coconut milk mixture and whisk until the gelatin is fully dissolved.
4. Strain the mixture through a fine-mesh sieve to remove any zest.
5. Pour the mixture into serving glasses or ramekins.
6. Refrigerate for at least 4 hours or until the panna cotta is set.
7. Garnish with fresh mint leaves before serving.

Nutritional Information:

Calories: 200 (per serving) | Protein: 2g | Fat: 18g | Net Carbs: 4g | Fiber: 0g

Key Benefits: Coconut milk provides healthy fats, while lime adds a refreshing citrus flavor.

Recipe Modification: Top with a dollop of whipped coconut cream and a sprinkle of toasted coconut.

VANILLA RICOTTA PARFAIT WITH BERRIES

Servings: 2-3

Prep Time: 10 minutes

Cook Time: 0 minutes

Ingredients:

- 1 cup whole milk ricotta cheese
- 2 tablespoons low-carb sweetener (such as erythritol)
- 1 teaspoon vanilla extract
- 1 cup mixed berries (strawberries, blueberries, raspberries)
- Chopped nuts (for garnish)

Instructions:

1. In a bowl, combine whole milk ricotta cheese, low-carb sweetener, and vanilla extract. Mix well.
2. Layer the ricotta mixture with mixed berries in serving glasses.
3. Repeat the layers until the glasses are filled.
4. Garnish with chopped nuts before serving.

Nutritional Information:

Calories: 200 (per serving) | Protein: 8g | Fat: 15g | Net Carbs: 6g | Fiber: 3g

Key Benefits: Ricotta cheese offers protein and calcium, while berries provide vitamins and antioxidants.

Recipe Modification: Drizzle with sugar-free chocolate sauce for extra indulgence.

COCONUT FLOUR LEMON BARS

Servings: 2-3

Prep Time: 15 minutes

Cook Time: 25 minutes

Ingredients:

- 1/2 cup coconut flour
- 1/4 cup low-carb sweetener (such as erythritol)
- 1/2 cup unsalted butter, melted
- 4 large eggs
- 1/4 cup fresh lemon juice
- 1 tablespoon lemon zest
- 1 teaspoon vanilla extract
- Pinch of salt

Instructions:

1. Preheat the oven to 350°F (175°C) and grease a baking dish.
2. In a bowl, combine coconut flour, low-carb sweetener, and melted butter. Press into the bottom of the baking dish to form the crust.
3. In another bowl, whisk together eggs, fresh lemon juice, lemon zest, vanilla extract, and a pinch of salt.
4. Pour the lemon mixture over the crust and spread evenly.
5. Bake in the oven for about 20-25 minutes or until the edges are golden and the center is set.
6. Let the bars cool completely before slicing and serving.

Nutritional Information:

Calories: 150 (per serving) | Protein: 4g | Fat: 12g | Net Carbs: 5g | Fiber: 3g

Key Benefits: Coconut flour provides fiber, while lemon adds refreshing flavor.

Recipe Modification: Dust with powdered erythritol for a touch of sweetness.

ALMOND BUTTER CHOCOLATE FUDGE

Servings: 2-3

Prep Time: 10 minutes

Cook Time: 0 minutes (plus chilling time)

Ingredients:

- 1/2 cup almond butter
- 1/4 cup coconut oil, melted
- 1/4 cup unsweetened cocoa powder
- 2 tablespoons low-carb sweetener (such as stevia)
- 1 teaspoon vanilla extract
- Pinch of salt

Instructions:

1. In a bowl, combine almond butter, melted coconut oil, unsweetened cocoa powder, low-carb sweetener, vanilla extract, and a pinch of salt. Mix well until smooth.
2. Pour the mixture into a lined baking dish and spread evenly.
3. Refrigerate for at least 2 hours or until the fudge is firm.
4. Cut into squares before serving.

Nutritional Information:

Calories: 150 (per serving) | Protein: 4g | Fat: 12g | Net Carbs: 4g | Fiber: 3g

Key Benefits: Almond butter provides protein and healthy fats, while cocoa powder offers antioxidants.

Recipe Modification: Top with a sprinkle of flaky sea salt for a gourmet touch.

PUMPKIN SPICE CHEESECAKE BITES

Servings: 2-3

Prep Time: 15 minutes

Cook Time: 25 minutes

Ingredients:

- 1 cup cream cheese, softened
- 1/2 cup canned pumpkin puree
- 1/4 cup low-carb sweetener (such as erythritol)
- 1 large egg
- 1 teaspoon pumpkin spice mix
- 1 teaspoon vanilla extract

Instructions:

1. Preheat the oven to 325°F (160°C) and line a mini muffin tin with paper liners.
2. In a bowl, beat cream cheese, canned pumpkin puree, low-carb sweetener, egg, pumpkin spice mix, and vanilla extract until smooth.
3. Spoon the mixture into the mini muffin tin, filling each cup almost to the top.
4. Bake in the oven for about 20-25 minutes or until the cheesecake bites are set.
5. Let them cool completely before removing from the tin.

Nutritional Information:

Calories: 150 (per serving) | Protein: 4g | Fat: 12g | Net Carbs: 5g | Fiber: 1g

Key Benefits: Pumpkin puree offers vitamins and fiber, while cream cheese provides richness.

Recipe Modification: Sprinkle with a touch of cinnamon before serving.

MIXED BERRY CRUMBLE

Servings: 2-3

Prep Time: 15 minutes

Cook Time: 25 minutes

Ingredients:

- 2 cups mixed berries (strawberries, blueberries, raspberries)
- 1 tablespoon low-carb sweetener (such as erythritol)
- 1 teaspoon lemon juice
- 1/2 cup almond flour
- 1/4 cup chopped pecans
- 2 tablespoons unsalted butter, melted
- 1/2 teaspoon cinnamon
- Pinch of salt

Instructions:

1. Preheat the oven to 350°F (175°C) and grease a baking dish.
2. In a bowl, combine mixed berries, low-carb sweetener, and lemon juice. Toss to coat the berries.
3. Spread the berry mixture in the bottom of the baking dish.
4. In another bowl, mix almond flour, chopped pecans, melted butter, cinnamon, and a pinch of salt until crumbly.
5. Sprinkle the almond flour mixture over the berries.
6. Bake in the oven for about 20-25 minutes or until the topping is golden and the berries are bubbly.
7. Let the crumble cool slightly before serving.

Nutritional Information:

Calories: 150 (per serving) | Protein: 4g | Fat: 12g | Net Carbs: 6g | Fiber: 4g

Key Benefits: Berries offer vitamins and antioxidants, while almond flour provides a nutty flavor.

Recipe Modification: Serve with a dollop of whipped cream or coconut cream.

CHOCOLATE AVOCADO MOUSSE

Servings: 2-3

Prep Time: 10 minutes

Cook Time: 0 minutes

Ingredients:

- 2 ripe avocados
- 1/4 cup unsweetened cocoa powder
- 1/4 cup low-carb sweetener (such as erythritol)
- 1 teaspoon vanilla extract
- Pinch of salt
- Fresh berries (for garnish)

Instructions:

1. In a blender or food processor, combine ripe avocados, cocoa powder, low-carb sweetener, vanilla extract, and a pinch of salt.
2. Blend until smooth and creamy, scraping down the sides as needed.
3. Divide the mousse into serving dishes and refrigerate for at least 1 hour to set.
4. Garnish with fresh berries before serving.

Nutritional Information:

Calories: 150 (per serving) | Protein: 2g | Fat: 12g | Net Carbs: 6g | Fiber: 4g

Key Benefits: Avocados offer healthy fats and vitamins, while cocoa powder provides antioxidants.

Recipe Modification: Top with chopped nuts for extra texture.

COCONUT CHIA SEED POPSICLES

Servings: 2-3

Prep Time: 10 minutes

Freeze Time: 4 hours (or overnight)

Ingredients:

- 1 cup unsweetened coconut milk
- 2 tablespoons chia seeds
- 2 tablespoons low-carb sweetener (such as stevia)
- 1/2 teaspoon vanilla extract

Instructions:

1. In a bowl, whisk together unsweetened coconut milk, chia seeds, low-carb sweetener, and vanilla extract.
2. Let the mixture sit for about 10 minutes to allow the chia seeds to absorb the liquid.
3. Pour the mixture into Popsicle molds and insert sticks.
4. Freeze for at least 4 hours or until the popsicles are solid.
5. Run the molds under warm water to release the popsicles before serving.

Nutritional Information:

Calories: 100 (per serving) | Protein: 2g | Fat: 8g | Net Carbs: 4g | Fiber: 6g

Key Benefits: Chia seeds provide fiber and omega-3 fatty acids, while coconut milk adds creaminess.

Recipe Modification: Mix in some chopped dark chocolate before freezing.

RASPBERRY ALMOND THUMBPRINT COOKIES

Servings: 2-3

Prep Time: 15 minutes

Cook Time: 15 minutes

Ingredients:

- 1 cup almond flour
- 2 tablespoons low-carb sweetener (such as erythritol)
- 2 tablespoons unsalted butter, softened
- 1/4 cup sugar-free raspberry jam
- 1/4 teaspoon almond extract

Instructions:

1. Preheat the oven to 350°F (175°C) and line a baking sheet with parchment paper.
2. In a bowl, mix almond flour, low-carb sweetener, and softened butter until a dough forms.
3. Roll the dough into small balls and place them on the baking sheet.
4. Make a small indentation in the center of each ball using your thumb.
5. Fill each indentation with sugar-free raspberry jam.
6. Bake in the oven for about 12-15 minutes or until the cookies are golden.
7. Let the cookies cool on the baking sheet before transferring to a wire rack.

Nutritional Information:

Calories: 150 (per serving) | Protein: 4g | Fat: 12g | Net Carbs: 4g | Fiber: 2g

Key Benefits: Almond flour provides a nutty flavor and healthy fats, while raspberry jam adds sweetness.

Recipe Modification: Substitute the jam with other sugar-free fruit preserves.

CINNAMON ALMOND BAKED APPLES

Servings: 2-3

Prep Time: 15 minutes

Cook Time: 30 minutes

Ingredients:

- 2 large apples, cored and halved
- 2 tablespoons almond butter
- 2 tablespoons chopped almonds
- 1 tablespoon low-carb sweetener (such as erythritol)
- 1 teaspoon ground cinnamon
- Pinch of nutmeg

Instructions:

1. Preheat the oven to 350°F (175°C) and grease a baking dish.
2. Place the cored and halved apples in the baking dish.
3. In a bowl, mix almond butter, chopped almonds, low-carb sweetener, ground cinnamon, and a pinch of nutmeg.
4. Fill the center of each apple half with the almond mixture.
5. Bake in the oven for about 25-30 minutes or until the apples are tender.
6. Serve the baked apples warm.

Nutritional Information:

Calories: 150 (per serving) | Protein: 4g | Fat: 10g | Net Carbs: 8g | Fiber: 6g

Key Benefits: Apples offer fiber and vitamins, while almonds provide healthy fats.

Recipe Modification: Top with a dollop of Greek yogurt or whipped cream.

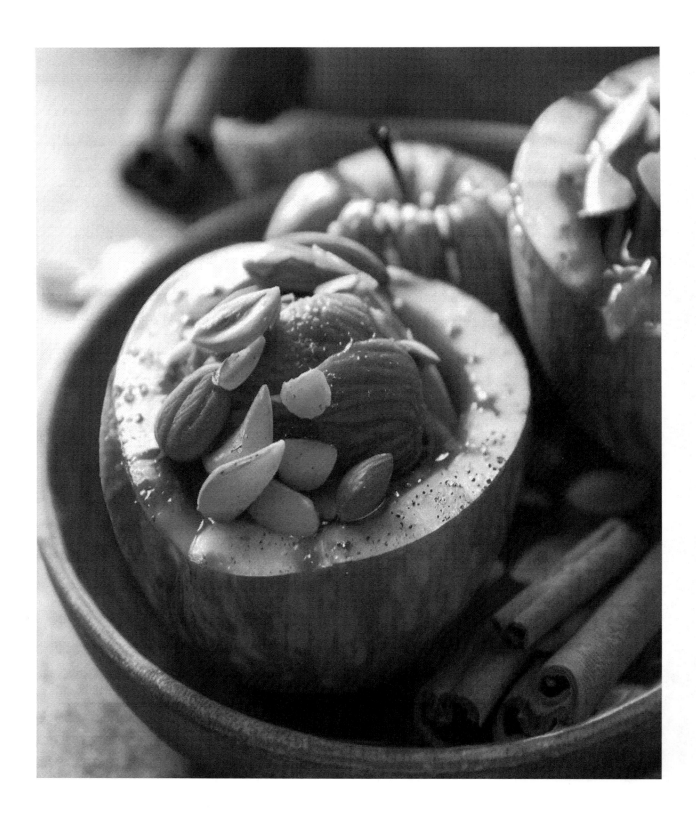

CHAPTER TWO: 28-DAY MEAL PLAN

WEEK 1

DAY	BREAKFAST	LUNCH	DINNER
1	Avocado and Bacon Breakfast Bowl	Zucchini Noodles with Pesto	Stuffed Bell Peppers
2	Cauliflower Crust Pizza	Greek Zucchini Boats	Creamy Garlic Parmesan Chicken
3	Keto Breakfast Burrito Bowl	Green Bean and Cherry Tomato Salad	Coconut Lime Panna Cotta
4	Spaghetti Squash Carbonara	Mediterranean Grilled Chicken Salad	Cabbage Stir-Fry with Ground Pork
5	Mixed Nuts and Cheese Platter	Chicken and Avocado Lettuce Wraps	Baked Salmon with Cauliflower Rice
6	Cinnamon Almond Baked Apples	Spaghetti Squash with Pesto and Cherry Tomatoes	Zucchini Noodles with Pesto and Grilled Shrimp
7	Chocolate Avocado Mousse	Greek Salad with Grilled Chicken	Cauliflower Crust Pizza with Salad

WEEK 2

DAY	BREAKFAST	LUNCH	DINNER
8	Baked Salmon with Asparagus and Lemon	Cauliflower and Broccoli Casserole	Zucchini Noodles with Pesto
9	Coconut Chia Seed Popsicles	Green Bean and Cherry Tomato Salad	Almond Butter Chocolate Fudge
10	Coconut Flour Lemon Bars	Spiced Cabbage and Carrot Slaw	Coconut Lime Panna Cotta
11	Mixed Nuts and Cheese Platter	Chicken and Avocado Lettuce Wraps	Grilled Lemon Herb Chicken with Asparagus
12	Mixed Berry Chia Seed Pudding	Spaghetti Squash with Pesto and Cherry Tomatoes	Baked Salmon with Cauliflower Rice
13	Low-Carb Breakfast Burrito	Greek Salad with Grilled Chicken	Zucchini Noodles with Pesto and Grilled Shrimp
14	Chocolate Avocado Mousse	Roasted Eggplant with Tahini Drizzle	Cauliflower Crust Pizza with Salad

	WEEK 3		
15	Creamy Garlic Parmesan Chicken	Spiced Cabbage and Carrot Slaw	Mixed Berry Crumble
16	Coconut Chia Seed Popsicles	Green Bean and Cherry Tomato Salad	Almond Butter Chocolate Fudge
17	Coconut Flour Lemon Bars	Chicken and Avocado Lettuce Wraps	Coconut Lime Panna Cotta
18	Pumpkin Spice Cheesecake Bites	Spaghetti Squash with Pesto and Cherry Tomatoes	Grilled Lemon Herb Chicken with Asparagus
19	Mixed Berry Chia Seed Pudding	Greek Salad with Grilled Chicken	Baked Salmon with Cauliflower Rice
20	Cinnamon Almond Baked Apples	Roasted Eggplant with Tahini Drizzle	Zucchini Noodles with Pesto and Grilled Shrimp
21	Chocolate Avocado Mousse	Chicken and Avocado Lettuce Wraps	Cauliflower Crust Pizza with Salad
	WEEK 4		
22	Vanilla Ricotta Parfait with Berries	Spiced Cabbage and Carrot Slaw	Mixed Nuts And Cheese Platter
23	Coconut Chia Seed Popsicles	Green Bean and Cherry Tomato Salad	Almond Butter Chocolate Fudge
24	Coconut Flour Lemon Bars	Spaghetti Squash with Pesto and Cherry Tomatoes	Coconut Lime Panna Cotta
25	Pumpkin Spice Cheesecake Bites	Chicken and Avocado Lettuce Wraps	Grilled Lemon Herb Chicken with Asparagus
26	Mixed Berry Chia Seed Pudding	Greek Salad with Grilled Chicken	Baked Salmon with Cauliflower Rice
27	Keto Breakfast Burrito Bowl	Roasted Eggplant with Tahini Drizzle	Zucchini Noodles with Pesto and Grilled Shrimp
28	Chocolate Avocado Mousse	Chicken and Avocado Lettuce Wraps	Cauliflower Crust Pizza with Salad

NOTE:

Feel free to adjust the meal plan based on your preferences and dietary needs. This plan incorporates a variety of flavors and ingredients while adhering to the principles of the Atkins Diet.

7-DAY WEIGHT LOSS EXERCISE PLAN

Incorporating regular exercise into your Atkins Diet journey can enhance your weight loss efforts, improve your overall health, and increase your energy levels. Here's a 7-day exercise plan designed to complement the Atkins Diet for beginners:

Day 1: Cardio Kickstart

- Warm-up: 5 minutes of light jogging or brisk walking.
- Main Exercise: 20-30 minutes of moderate-intensity cardio, such as cycling, swimming, or brisk walking.
- Cool-down: 5-10 minutes of stretching.

Day 2: Total Body Strength

- Warm-up: 5 minutes of light cardio.
- Main Exercise: Perform bodyweight exercises like squats, push-ups, lunges, and planks. Aim for 3 sets of 12-15 reps for each exercise.
- Cool-down: 5-10 minutes of stretching.

Day 3: Active Rest and Flexibility

- Engage in light activities like gentle yoga, stretching, or a leisurely walk to promote flexibility and relaxation.

Day 4: Interval Training

- Warm-up: 5 minutes of light cardio.
- Main Exercise: Alternate between 1 minute of high-intensity exercise (such as sprinting or jumping jacks) and 1-2 minutes of low-intensity recovery. Repeat for 20-25 minutes.
- Cool-down: 5-10 minutes of stretching.

Day 5: Lower Body Focus

- Warm-up: 5 minutes of light cardio.
- Main Exercise: Perform exercises targeting your lower body, such as squats, lunges, leg press, and calf raises. Aim for 3 sets of 12-15 reps for each exercise.
- Cool-down: 5-10 minutes of stretching.

Day 6: Active Rest and Outdoor Activity

- Engage in an outdoor activity you enjoy, such as hiking, biking, or playing a sport. This is an opportunity to have fun while staying active.

Day 7: Core and Flexibility

- Warm-up: 5 minutes of light cardio.
- Main Exercise: Focus on core-strengthening exercises like planks, Russian twists, and bicycle crunches. Perform 3 sets of 12-15 reps for each exercise.
- Cool-down: 5-10 minutes of stretching.

Important Tips:

1. Listen to your body. If an exercise feels uncomfortable or painful, modify or skip it.
2. Stay hydrated before, during, and after your workouts.
3. Incorporate a mix of cardiovascular, strength, and flexibility exercises for a well-rounded routine.
4. Gradually increase the intensity and duration of your workouts as you become more comfortable.
5. Consult a healthcare professional before starting any new exercise program, especially if you have underlying health concerns.

Remember, consistency is key. By combining regular exercise with the Atkins Diet's principles, you're creating a holistic approach to achieving your weight loss goals and improving your overall well-being.

CONCLUSION

Congratulations on completing your journey through the "Atkins Diet Cookbook for Beginners." This comprehensive guide has provided you with the essential tools, knowledge, and delicious recipes to embark on a successful and sustainable path toward improved health and weight management. As you reflect on the information shared and the recipes discovered, let's recap the key takeaways from your journey:

Embracing the Atkins Diet:

You've gained an understanding of the Atkins Diet's fundamental principles, including its four phases. From minimizing carbohydrates and prioritizing protein to incorporating healthy fats and fiber, the Atkins Diet promotes a balanced approach to nutrition that can lead to steady weight loss and overall wellness.

Meal Planning and Preparation:

The art of meal planning and prepping has been demystified. Armed with a carefully designed 28-day meal plan, you've learned how to create a shopping list that includes lean meats, nutrient-rich vegetables, low-carb fruits, and essential pantry staples. These practices are instrumental in maintaining dietary consistency and supporting your weight loss goals.

Delightful and Nutritious Recipes:

With a wide range of recipes for breakfast, lunch, dinner, snacks, and desserts, you've discovered that the Atkins Diet doesn't mean sacrificing flavor or variety. From avocado and bacon breakfast bowls to zucchini noodles with pesto, each dish has been carefully crafted to align with the diet's principles while satisfying your taste buds.

Exercise for Enhanced Results:

Complementing your dietary efforts, the 7-day exercise plan has provided you with a balanced mix of cardiovascular, strength, and flexibility exercises. This plan not only supports weight loss but also boosts your energy levels and overall well-being. Remember, consistency in your workouts, coupled with the Atkins Diet, can bring about lasting positive changes.

Mindful Progress and Beyond:

As you move forward, keep in mind that the Atkins Diet is not just a temporary solution but a lifestyle choice. Embrace the concept of transitioning between phases as your weight loss journey progresses. Stay open to trying new recipes and foods, and always prioritize nutrient-rich options. Remember that a holistic approach to health includes not only what you eat but also how you move and care for yourself.

By integrating the knowledge and practices you've gained from this cookbook, you're equipped with the tools to achieve and maintain a healthier lifestyle. The "Atkins Diet Cookbook for Beginners" has laid a solid foundation for you to build upon, guiding you toward better health, increased vitality, and improved confidence. As you continue your journey, don't forget that patience, dedication, and consistency are your greatest allies. Celebrate every milestone, no matter how small, and keep moving forward on your path to wellness.

BONUS: WEIGHT LOSS JOURNAL

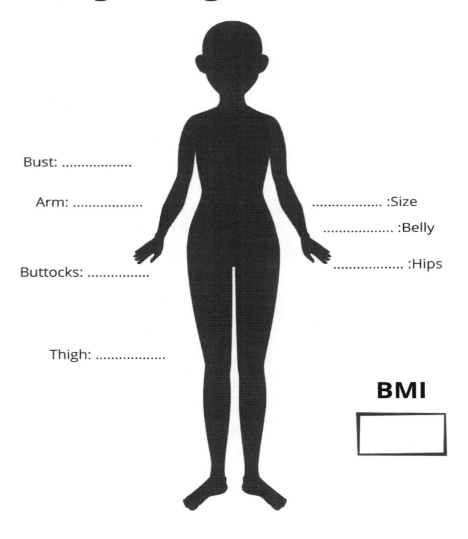

111 | Atkins Diet Cookbook for Beginners

The first day

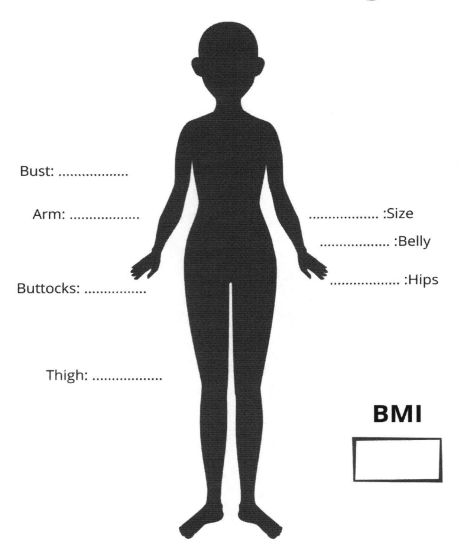

Bust: ....

Arm: ....

.... :Size

.... :Belly

.... :Hips

Buttocks: ....

Thigh: ....

BMI

Weight: ....

Day n° ....   Weight: ....

My energy intake

Breakfast: ....   Lunch: ....
....
....

Dinner: ....   Snacks: ....
....
....

Details   *My energy expenses*

                                                    Kcal:

Sleep: .... ▭

                                         .... ▭

Protein: .... ▭

                                         .... ▭

Hydration: .... ▭

                                         .... ▭

Motivation: ☺ ☹   .... ▭
              ○ ○

📝 **Notes:** ....
....
....
....
....

Day n° .... Weight: ....

My energy intake

Breakfast: .... Lunch: ....
....
....

Dinner: .... Snacks: ....
....
....

Details *My energy expenses*

Kcal:

Sleep: .... ☐

.... ☐

Protein: .... ☐

.... ☐

Hydration: .... ☐

Motivation: ☺ ☹ .... ☐
○ ○ .... ☐

📝 **Notes:** ....
....
....
....

Day n° ....   Weight: ....

My energy intake

Breakfast: ....   Lunch: ....

....

....

Dinner: ....   Snacks: ....

....

....

Details   *My energy expenses*

                                              Kcal:

Sleep: .... [ ]

                                              .... [ ]

Protein: .... [ ]

                                              .... [ ]

Hydration: .... [ ]

                                              .... [ ]

Motivation: ☺ ☹   .... [ ]
             ○ ○

📝 Notes: ....

....

....

....

Day n° .... Weight: ....

My energy intake

Breakfast: .... Lunch: ....
....
....

Dinner: .... Snacks: ....
....
....

Details *My energy expenses*

Kcal:

Sleep: .... ▭

.... ▭

Protein: .... ▭

.... ▭

Hydration: .... ▭

Motivation: ☺ ☹ .... ▭

.... ▭

📝 **Notes:** ....
....
....
....
....

Day n° ....   Weight: ....

My energy intake

Breakfast: ....   Lunch: ....
....
....

Dinner: ....   Snacks: ....
....
....

Details   *My energy expenses*
                                                     Kcal:

Sleep: .... ▭

                                           .... ▭

Protein: .... ▭

                                           .... ▭

Hydration: .... ▭

                                           .... ▭

Motivation: ☺ ☹   .... ▭
            ○ ○

📝 **Notes:** ....
....
....
....
....

Day n° ....   Weight: ....

My energy intake

Breakfast: ....   Lunch: ....
....
....

Dinner: ....   Snacks: ....
....
....

Details   *My energy expenses*

                                                                      Kcal:

Sleep: .... ☐

                                              .... ☐

Protein: .... ☐

                                              .... ☐

Hydration: .... ☐

                                              .... ☐

Motivation: ☺ ☹   .... ☐
             ○   ○

📝 **Notes:** ....
....
....
....
....

Day n° ....   Weight: ....

My energy intake

Breakfast: ....   Lunch: ....
....
....

Dinner: ....   Snacks: ....
....
....

Details   *My energy expenses*
                                                              Kcal:

Sleep: .... [ ]

                                                 .... [ ]

Protein: .... [ ]

                                                 .... [ ]

Hydration: .... [ ]

                                                 .... [ ]

Motivation: ☺ ☹   .... [ ]
                    ○ ○

📝 **Notes:** ....
....
....
....
....

Day n° .... Weight: ....

My energy intake

Breakfast: .... Lunch: ....
....
....

Dinner: .... Snacks: ....
....
....

Details

Sleep: ....

Protein: ....

Hydration: ....

Motivation: 🙂 ☹

My energy expenses

Kcal:

.... [ ]
.... [ ]
.... [ ]
.... [ ]
.... [ ]
.... [ ]
.... [ ]

📝 Notes: ....
....
....
....
....

Day n° ....   Weight: ....

My energy intake

Breakfast: ....   Lunch: ....
....
....

Dinner: ....   Snacks: ....
....
....

Details   *My energy expenses*

                                                                                            Kcal:

Sleep: .... ▭

Protein: .... ▭

Hydration: .... ▭

Motivation: ☺ ☹   .... ▭
                ○ ○   .... ▭
                                                                .... ▭

📝 **Notes:** ....
....
....
....
....

Day n° ....   Weight: ....

My energy intake

Breakfast: ....   Lunch: ....
....
....

Dinner: ....   Snacks: ....
....
....

Details   *My energy expenses*

                                                                                     Kcal:

Sleep: .... [ ]

                                       .... [ ]

Protein: .... [ ]

                                       .... [ ]

Hydration: .... [ ]

                                       .... [ ]

Motivation: ☺ ☹   .... [ ]
                 ○ ○

📝 **Notes:** ....
....
....
....
....

We've sweated over stovetops, danced with ingredients, and even managed to keep our aprons mostly stain-free (well, mostly).

Now that you've journeyed through "Atkins Diet Cookbook for Beginners" why not sprinkle a little seasoning of your thoughts in the form of a review? It's like leaving a food critic's note but without the fancy hat! Your feedback adds the secret ingredient to our future creations, and who knows, maybe we'll even name a recipe after you (we can't promise that, but it's a fun thought). So, whether you're a gourmet guru or a kitchen newbie, drop us a review, and let's keep the flavor train rolling.

Thanks a bunch, and remember, reviews are calorie-free and always in good taste!

[Emily M. Wilson]

Made in the USA
Las Vegas, NV
04 January 2024

83898153R00068